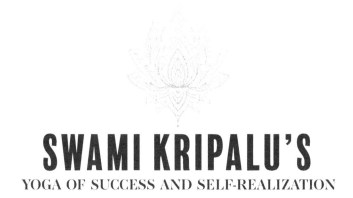

SWAMI KRIPALU'S
YOGA OF SUCCESS AND SELF-REALIZATION

SWAMI KRIPALU'S
YOGA OF SUCCESS AND SELF-REALIZATION

RICHARD FAULDS

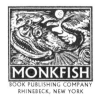

MONKFISH
BOOK PUBLISHING COMPANY
RHINEBECK, NEW YORK

Swami Kripalu's Yoga of Success and Self-Realization © copyright 2025 by Richard Faulds

All rights reserved. No part of this book may be used or reproduced in any manner without the consent of the publisher except for in critical articles or reviews. Contact the publisher for information.

The archival materials upon which this book is based are used by permission of Kripalu Center for Yoga & Health, Stockbridge, MA, www.kripalu.org. All the photographs appearing in this book, unless otherwise noted, including its cover are from the archives of Umesh Eric Baldwin and reprinted here with his permission. For a wealth of photographs and information about the life and teachings of Swami Kripalu, visit www.swamikripalvananda.org.

Paperback ISBN 978-1-958972-70-0
eBook ISBN 978-1-958972-71-7

Library of Congress Cataloging-in-Publication Data

Names: Faulds, Richard, author.
Title: Swami Kripalu's yoga of success and self-realization / Richard
    Faulds.
Description: Rhinebeck, New York : Monkfish Book Publishing Company, [2025]
Identifiers: LCCN 2024062139 (print) | LCCN 2024062140 (ebook) | ISBN
    9781958972700 (paperback) | ISBN 9781958972717 (ebook)
Subjects: LCSH: Yoga--Psychological aspects. | Kripalvanandji, Swami,
    1913-1981. | Self-realization--Religious aspects--Hinduism.
Classification: LCC BL1238.52 .F38 2025 (print) | LCC BL1238.52 (ebook) |
    DDC 294.5/436--dc23/eng/20250110
LC record available at https://lccn.loc.gov/2024062139
LC ebook record available at https://lccn.loc.gov/2024062140

Book and cover design by Colin Rolfe

Monkfish Book Publishing Company
22 East Market Street, Suite 304
Rhinebeck, New York 12572
(845) 876-4861
monkfishpublishing.com

For all those who did not have the opportunity given me to meet Swami Kripalu, even if only once.

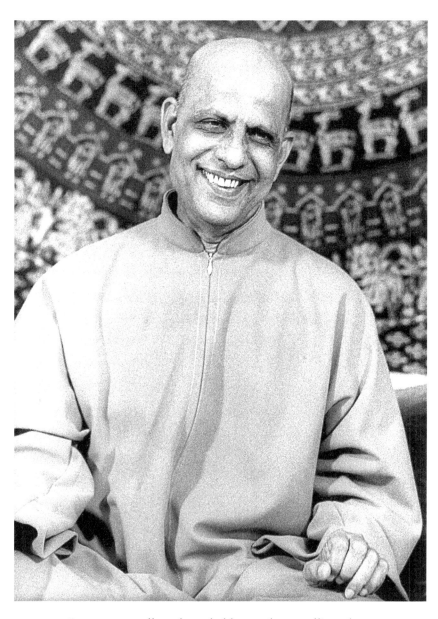

*I encourage all my householder students, telling them:
Establish yourself like a sun in the solar system of society.*
—SWAMI KRIPALU

CONTENTS

Note to the Reader ... ix

PART ONE
Introducing Yoga, Swami Kripalu, and the Householder Path

| Chapter 1 | Life Sketch of Swami Kripalu | 7 |
| Chapter 2 | The Epiphany at the Heart of this Book | 10 |

PART TWO
Grasp the Essence of Yoga

Chapter 3	Gift of the Sages	29
Chapter 4	Empowerment through Self Discovery	39
Chapter 5	Purushartha: The Four Aims of Life	53
Chapter 6	Svadharma: Your Life Purpose	69
Chapter 7	Sadharana Dharma: The Ethical Principles Applicable to All	84
Chapter 8	Sanatana Dharma: A Yoga-Based Life Path	96
Chapter 9	Sanatana Dharma in Practice	106
Chapter 10	How Yoga Works	116
Chapter 11	A Map to Guide Your Journey	125

PART THREE
The Foundational Practices

Chapter 12	The Seed Disposition	145
Chapter 13	A Discipline of Daily Practice	148
Chapter 14	Healthy Living	157
Chapter 15	Love in the Family	172
Chapter 16	The Importance of Character Building	183

Chapter 17	Character Building Through Practicing the Opposite	190
Chapter 18	Mantra Yoga	207
Chapter 19	Mantra Yoga in Practice	221
Chapter 20	Skillfulness in Action	235

| Afterword | | 245 |
| Acknowledgments | | 247 |

Appendix 1:	The Character-Building Principles of Yama and Niyama	249
Appendix 2:	Teaching Stories	281
Appendix 3:	Instructional Handouts	313

NOTE TO THE READER

Like the Indian sages in whose footsteps he walked, Swami Kripalu taught yoga as a wisdom tradition in which disciples maintain a close personal relationship to their guru and demonstrate their fitness to receive each level of its esoteric curriculum through the intensity of their study, practice, and devotion. He adopted this approach for an important reason, as the single-minded dedication it required was meant to bring forth the best from his top students to preserve yoga's spiritual depth and transformative potency. Yet this approach also had a downside in that it failed to make the full scope of his teachings accessible to a multitude of seekers unable to join his circle of intimates.

This book presents Swami Kripalu's teachings in a contemporary framework that any reader can understand and put into practice. While I've provided a narrative text, its chief content is the extensive body of quotations, excerpts, and teaching stories that remain as close as possible to his actual words. Every effort has been made to retain his distinctive voice and subtlety of expression. The quotes have been ordered and edited to compliment the text sections in which they appear. To convey a whole message on a particular topic, it was often necessary to combine material from different sources and express them in a single narrative. Rather than academic literalness, I strove to present his guidance in a straightforward fashion true to the original.

It's important to know that all quotations drawn from Swami Kripalu's legacy of published works, scholarly discourses, transcribed talks, and personal correspondence are presented in *italics*. That includes the epigraphs that open each chapter, the segregated sections interspersed throughout the text, and margin quotes. I tried to moderate my use of the Sanskrit terms that permeate the original materials, defining important ones for readers eager to learn more, while respecting those who want things said in plain English. In places where Swami Kripalu's name is repeated often in my narrative text, it is shortened to SK for ease of reading.

This is the second of three books researched and written in the dozen years since I retired as a staff member of Kripalu Center for Yoga & Health. It follows *Dharma Then Moksha: The Untold Story of Swami Kripalu*, an illustrated recounting of his remarkable life that begins with my experience of meeting Swami Kripalu shortly before his death in 1981, an encounter that set me on the path of yoga just as I was crossing the threshold into adulthood. This book continues the series and starts out explaining how my youthful hunch that his householder path had unknown possibilities matured into a surprising discovery. The third and final book will be *Swami Kripalu's Ladder of Yoga* (forthcoming from Monkfish). It retraces the efforts of myself and others to progress along this path into the depths of yoga. While *Dharma Then Moksha* is a stand-alone work, notations appear throughout the subsequent two books to show the close correspondence between how Swami Kripalu lived and what he taught, in effect making the series a trilogy.

After completing my research, I can say that Swami Kripalu taught the principles of yoga with great precision. His talks and stories are riddled with shorthand references to other teaching areas that show how these principles fit together and apply across multiple stages of yoga. By catching these references in specific passages, I was often able to discern the full meaning of a particular point he was making and place it in the context of his overall curriculum. It is this kind of analysis that allowed me to spotlight matters central to today's practitioners, and bring forth facets of his teachings that have never before appeared in print. While alive and teaching masterfully, he probably would not have appreciated me or anyone interpreting his words. But after his death, it became necessary for someone familiar with his life and yoga to do this editorial cross-referencing to produce a reliable synthesis of his teachings. As to the quality of my work, I can only say it was carefully done and direct readers wanting greater specificity to his verbatim teachings.

In the four decades since meeting Swami Kripalu, I've practiced yoga drawing on many resources but always returning to his teachings as the lantern needed to navigate my way through whatever new and unknown landscape I happened to be passing. Looking back, it's my belief that anyone can apply the principles he taught to improve their health, catalyze psychological growth, and channel their energies into a successful outer life while also experiencing high levels of inner awakening. May this book be a helpful companion on your journey.

RICHARD FAULDS
Greenville, Virginia

PART ONE

INTRODUCING YOGA, SWAMI KRIPALU, AND THE HOUSEHOLDER PATH

Yoga has many definitions but for now let us consider it to mean "solution." We are all striving to avoid suffering and satisfy our needs and desires. Yoga provides the true tools of self-development that enable us to do both. Wherever yoga is practiced systematically, good health and fulfillment naturally follow.

The ancient Indian sages discovered things about the body and mind that science is only now beginning to understand. These discoveries occurred in the midst of their religious quest to access the singular power and intelligence they speculated must lie at the root of existence. In trying to find out firsthand if the diversity of the natural world has its source in an unseen inner unity, the sages were compelled to optimize the functioning of all their faculties. It was this impetus that led them to develop a wide array of contemplative techniques that evolved over many centuries and were eventually systematized into the postures, breathing exercises, relaxation protocols, and meditation methods that we know today as yoga.

As science studies these techniques, yoga is proving its effectiveness. Alongside the gains in strength, flexibility, coordination, endurance, bone density, and respiratory function commonly associated with physical fitness, yoga practitioners report a host of other benefits that a robust body of medical research is steadily validating. This includes stronger digestion; deeper sleep; more energy; elevated mood; greater ease of movement; an appetite for healthier foods; fewer headaches; heightened self-awareness; sharper attentional focus and mindfulness; better concentration; higher self-esteem; increased empathy; an improved ability to regulate emotions, manage stress, and cope with chronic pain; and access to a wide range of rejuvenating mind states that inject life with meaning and purpose. Finding all these traits in long-term practitioners at significantly higher rates than the normal population, the scientists researching yoga's efficacy tout its ability to increase global human functioning.

Yoga has gone viral for a good reason: it works. In America alone, there are over 36 million people practicing regularly and sticking with it because their time on the yoga mat makes them more vital, creative, resilient, and masterful in their lives. This number would have to be multiplied many times to assess the actual scale and scope of the movement, as yoga has truly become a worldwide phenomenon.

The Indian sages who originated yoga explained how it works in simple terms. An early text called the Bhagavad Gita,[1] says: "Yoga is a harmony. Not for one who eats too much, or for one who eats too little. Not for one who sleeps too little, or for one who sleeps too much. A harmony in eating and resting, in sleeping and keeping awake, a skillfulness in whatever one does. This is the yoga that grants deliverance from the oppression of pain." The sages were well aware the naturalness they were describing was not easy to come by. That's why yoga involves a progressive training in which students learn how to integrate the body and mind, fine tuning all the systems that support health and effective functioning.

Once established, the sages saw this healthy state of mind-body harmony as the fertile ground in which the seeds of our higher capacities can sprout and blossom. The Gita goes on to declare that a yogi practicing this harmony will soon know peace of mind, feel an upwelling of joy in the heart, find fulfillment in skillfully discharging their duties in life, and obtain a liberating vision of the highest truth. This optimistic view of yoga's ability to catalyze positive change is mirrored in many traditional texts and borne out by the experience of practitioners today, who discover

---

[1] Scholars date the earliest versions of the Bhagavad Gita to 400 BCE. This quote is from chapter 6, verses 16-17. The Yoga Sutra is another authoritative text circa 200 CE that explains how yoga practice eliminates mental turbulence so reality can be seen clearly—see 1:2 and 1:3. Still later is the Mgendra Tantra written between 600-1000 CE, which explains how yoga enables a person to gain control of their faculties and attain self-mastery—see 1.1.17.

that yoga's physical benefits readily spill over into personal and spiritual growth.

> *Yoga harmonizes the body and mind. The breath flows easily in and out, and the senses grow calm. Everything comes together and unites in one place. All the tools of yoga are intended to do this. It's much like tuning a radio to eliminate the static that prevents it from working properly. Absent this attunement, a person cannot experience real peace and joy. Only after the body and mind are harmonized and true health is experienced can the deeper attainments of yoga come forth.*

While helpful guidance to practitioners, the sage's generalizations offer little assistance to researchers tasked with explaining how yoga works in the rigorous terminology of physiology, biochemistry, and neuroscience. After a century of effort, science has proven that yoga offers a lengthy list of discrete benefits, and that regular practice is positively correlated to the cornerstones of a healthy lifestyle including wholesome eating, exercise adherence, lower body mass index, better mental health, less insomnia and sleep disturbance, and reduced substance/medication use. But the way the body and mind function and interact is exceedingly intricate, as reflected in the fact that science has yet to unravel the way everyday drugs like aspirin and ibuprofen operate. While considerable knowledge has been gained, a comprehensive explanation of how yoga works its magic has been hard to nail down. For those interested in the technicalities, the current thinking is summarized in the sidebar.

HOW YOGA WORKS

Science began studying yoga in the 1920s, but only recently has a critical mass of research come together in the fields of yoga, meditation, and mindfulness to suggest its real range of benefits and start to shed light on the mechanisms through which it works. Some of the studies cited below were performed or funded by Kripalu Center, an early leader in the field of yoga research.
- Relieves stress by reducing psycho-physiological arousal and activating the relaxation response to slow heart rate,

lower blood pressure, optimize hormone levels such as noradrenalin and cortisol, improve the quality of sleep, and decrease the incidence of back pain and other stress-related symptoms and behaviors.
- Elevates mood and eases anxiety/depression by improving stress regulation in ways that hike GABA levels and otherwise positively shift brain neurochemistry.
- Improves bone density and increases "bone quality," which is not measured by typical bone density scans but is important to resisting fractures.
- Enhances immune function and increases resistance to viral and possibly other infections.
- Shifts the activity of our cognitive attentional network away from its default mode of mental wandering and returns it more rapidly to a mindful and productive focus that enhances stress regulation, moderates emotions, and leads to less mood disturbance.
- Reduces the symptoms of ADHD in children and adolescents.
- Increases cerebral blood flow to beneficial brain regions that raise pain tolerance, improve our capacity to monitor mental attention, and over time preserve functional brain architecture, slowing the natural decline in fluid intelligence associated with aging.
- Decreases cerebral blood flow to brain regions involved in triggering stress and emotional reactivity such as the amygdala.
- Increases gray matter density and distribution in ways that support learning, memory processing, emotional regulation, self-awareness, and perspective taking.
- Raises mind-body awareness, which leads to dietary and lifestyle choices that avoid behaviors and risk factors known to undermine health and well-being.
- Shifts genomic expression to activate genes associated with insulin secretion and the mitochondrial function essential to energy metabolism, while inhibiting genes

associated with inflammatory response and stress-related pathways.
- Slows aging at the cellular level by protecting telomeres, the tiny caps on the end of chromosomes, which are believed to factor into healthy longevity.
- Turns off the neural circuitry that causes us to identify ourselves as separate and insular individuals, while enhancing the circuitry that supports mental focus and concentration. This combination enables us to vividly experience ourselves as empathically connected with everything around us and part of something greater than our individual selves. These "unitive experiences" act like catalysts, positively transforming our attitudes and worldview, and imbuing life with a greater sense of meaning, purpose, and spirituality.

The science of yoga is a subject dear to me. The mind affects the body, and the body affects the mind. That is the basic principle, but it cannot be proved by arguments alone. Experiments are indispensable. When an idea is proven with the help of a scientific experiment, it does not remain a mere idea but attains the status of truth. A physician giving a prescribed medication does not have to reveal its ingredients or explain how it was prepared. This is not necessary because the patient accepts science and is willing to take the medicine in order to get rid of the disease. Proving yoga's efficacy to such an extent would be of great benefit to many people, so it is my belief that all yogis should cooperate with scientists to test yoga properly.

If you are among the estimated 83 million Americans interested in trying yoga, you are probably looking for an exercise modality able to keep you physically fit, counter the negative effects of stress, uplevel your quotient of emotional and psychological wellness, stave off debilitating illness, and possibly deliver the boon of a spiritual experience. Even at this preliminary stage of research, the data is definitive that yoga is a wise choice.

Today's enthusiasts tend to see yoga as a mind-body practice that provides these and other tangible benefits, helping them live with greater zest and inner calm. The ancient sages saw yoga more broadly as a life path in which yoga practices are combined with a congruent set of philosophical and psychological principles, plus the cornerstone of a holistic lifestyle, to not only bestow health but actualize potentials in many areas. To them yoga was a way of living that could be relied upon to bring a practitioner what they saw as the two overarching goals of life: human fulfillment and spiritual freedom.[2]

Whether you're interested in yoga as a stand-alone practice or want to weave its elements into a holistic lifestyle, this book is a guide to reaping all the benefits that yoga has to offer. Rather than a substitute for a class or teacher, it's meant to complement both by providing the breadth and depth of instruction that today's fitness-oriented approaches often overlook. If you feel drawn to explore this time-tested path of self-development, here is a contemporary approach that is both true to the teachings of its originators and consistent with contemporary science.

> *Yoga is a path that can fulfill your worldly life and lead you into eternity. It is important to understand its core philosophy, which is very scientific in nature. The ancient sages who established yoga conducted experiments and found truths that even today are working with the same efficiency and effectiveness. To raise your own well-being and consciousness, you must do the experiments, but knowing the research they did and results they obtained will be of much interest and use to you.*

---

[2] Yoga's notion of spiritual freedom is twofold. First comes the freedom from suffering. That is followed by the freedom to act dynamically and express yourself creatively in a joyous life.

CHAPTER 1
LIFE SKETCH OF SWAMI KRIPALU

As a youth of nineteen, I had the opportunity to sit at the feet of a great man. As a yoga guru, he shone like the sun. For no reason known to me, this great guru loved me as a son and made me his chief disciple. It is with his blessing that I have set out to complete the cycle of yoga. I know it is only by his grace that I have come this far. At this point in my life, there is no attraction left for name or fame or wealth. I only want to go as far as the path of yoga can take me.

While born in the twentieth century, Swami Kripalu (1913-81) can rightly be counted among the yogic sages. The namesake of Kripalu Center for Yoga & Health, his life bridged the religious mysticism of ancient India with the secular and scientific West. Tragedy struck early when the untimely death of Swami Kripalu's father death plunged the family into debt. He grew up suffering poverty's many pains until age nineteen, when he met a teacher who initiated him into one of the oldest known schools of yoga. Practicing its teachings with uncommon zeal, he overcame his childhood adversity by distinguishing himself in the fields of literature and music. In midlife, he became a swami and relied upon these same teachings to achieve renown as an orator, educator, and social benefactor. Utilizing his fame to establish libraries, health clinics, vocational schools, and spiritual centers throughout western India, SK was recognized as one of the country's great humanitarian saints.

At the pinnacle of his outward success, Swami Kripalu experienced a profound energetic awakening that heralded a dramatic shift in his life. Relinquishing his role as a celebrated public figure, he devoted his last three decades to intensive kundalini yoga meditation and scriptural study, pursuing the end stages of yoga described in the traditional texts but seldom achieved by contemporary practitioners. It was near the end of this time that he came to America seeking a quiet place entirely out of the public eye to complete his practice. Arriving in 1977, he spent his final four years in residence at the original Kripalu Center facility in rural Pennsylvania before returning to India and dying only three months later in December 1981.

Although SK praised the efforts of today's scientists to solve the riddle of how yoga works, he knew their research was likely to continue for decades. In the meantime, he believed that yoga's guiding principles had already been articulated by its pioneering sages. Anyone able to put them into action could receive all their attendant benefits. To support that effort, he began work to distill the spectacularly diverse yoga tradition into a modern set of teachings designed to help students scale the ladder of human development to its upper rungs of self-actualization and Self-realization.

One of the dreams SK brought with him to America was the hope that his practice would culminate in the stable transcendental knowing praised by the Bhagavad Gita as the apex of yoga and these teachings would form the nucleus of a yoga university where everyone could come to learn the science of healthy living, character building, and spiritual awakening. This vision helped birth Kripalu Center and made it a beacon for all those wanting to explore life's deeper possibilities. Unfortunately, the effort to compile his teachings into a cogent curriculum was curtailed by his early death.

A tree must grow to its full height to give shade to others. In the same way, only a yogi who has truly reached to the highest can give yoga's message to the world. Although old enough to be your grandfather, I am still in seed form, and have come to America to continue my pilgrimage of yoga. I am very much pleased to meet you, and have faith that your love will be a great assistance in helping me complete my journey. Together may we all go all the way to God, that is my prayer and blessing.

Swami Kripalu had a special place in his heart for those students he called *my dear daughters and sons of America*. Incidents abound in which he went out of his way to ensure that his talks and writings were translated into English and made available *to continue the flow of knowledge started by Swami Vivekananda until yoga can be practiced properly and the distance between the spiritual sciences of India and the material sciences of the western world has been removed.*[1] May this book preserve the memory of Swami Kripalu in the only way he would have wanted, by inspiring individuals to discover the power of yoga through personal practice and keep the tradition of the Indian sages alive and evolving.

> *To study the physical universe of nature, scientists make the senses extrovert and take the support of instruments such as the microscope and telescope. To study that same universe's spiritual source, yogis make the senses introvert and take the support of postures, breath control, and meditation to increase their inner awareness. Western scientists may not understand the results of these yogic experiments, but they have been conducted in India for centuries, and there are scientific principles behind them. Material science has resulted in many surprising discoveries. When the airplane, radio, submarine, telephone and television were invented, people were spellbound and considered them miraculous. From the unbiased viewpoint of science, it is appropriate for modern scientists to consider the validity of yoga. These experiments are being conducted now in the United States, and I am confident that researchers will come to see the methods of yoga as integral parts of physical hygiene, anatomy, physiology, psychology, and medical science. It is my expectation and feeling that in one hundred years America will be a great center of yogic culture.*

---

[1] Swami Vivekananda was an Indian monk who traveled to Chicago in 1893 and gave a famous speech at the Parliament of World Religions. Afterward he toured the country delivering hundreds of lectures and is widely credited for introducing Hindu thought and yoga to Americans.

CHAPTER 2
THE EPIPHANY AT THE HEART OF THIS BOOK

Science knows little about those eureka moments when lightning strikes and innovative ideas emerge fully formed, but today's brain researchers are rapidly learning more. It now appears that epiphanies are not isolated events but the tail end of an integrated process. Faced with a complex problem, we draw upon the analytical left side of the brain to gather pertinent information. If the problem area is fraught with contradictions, this may take months, years, or even decades of painstaking investigation as we cognize an enormous amount of data. When gestation completes, the pattern recognition capacity of the right brain fires to reorganize the neural database, often in a moment of repose in which the analytical left brain is disengaged and we least expect it. An outmoded and incongruous way of beholding the world is replaced by a revelatory new interpretation of reality that removes some or all of the anomalies. It's against this backdrop of objective science that I want to share my personal story of one such epiphany.[1]

After three-and-a-half decades on the path of Kripalu Yoga, I stepped

---

[1] Hermann von Helmholtz (1821-94) was a pioneering German scientist and the first to describe epiphanies as a three-stage process of saturation, incubation, and illumination. Differences between the right and left hemispheres of the brain were noticed in the mid-1800s. In the 1970s, a simplistic model of the differences was put forth that remains a mainstay of pop psychology. While the bulk of this model has been discredited, more sophisticated analysis suggests that these hemispheric differences are significant and not only play a role in epiphanies but factor heavily in individual consciousness and collective culture. See the work of British psychiatrist Iain McGilchrist, especially *The Master and His Emissary: The Divided Brain and the Making of the Western World*.

away from my administrative role as Kripalu Center's lawyer to write a book on Swami Kripalu. I'd been awarded a generous two-year grant and my goal was straightforward: author a single volume that opened with a life sketch and closed with a restatement of his teachings targeted to meet the needs of today's practitioners. I knew this was no easy task. At times, SK described the yoga tradition as an ocean of disparate texts. This was an apt portrayal of his voluminous talks and writings too. In the thirty-five years since his death, no one had managed to condense the scope and scale of SK's teachings into a format that could be systematically practiced by anyone but those students who had known him personally. As a result, his valuable legacy languished.

India is the land of yoga's origin, where its practice has been carried out individually and collectively for thousands of years. Experienced yogis have always pondered their practice and offered critical evaluations of its results, so there is a sea of yogic literature that is very deep and also spreads far and wide. Without a boat in the form of a teacher, it is easy to drown in it.

Despite these difficulties, I accepted the grant as an opportunity to engage in the kind of depth exploration that had originally drawn me to the Kripalu community. It also positioned me to give back to a teaching lineage that had brought so many good things into my life. Having the luxury of time, I began by re-reading everything that Swami Kripalu had written or said that was available in English. This included a hard copy of Kripalu Center's archives, over a thousand pages of his talks translated on the spot and transcribed soon afterwards. Then I branched out to read everything that others had written about him or his teachings. I balanced all this study with an equal amount of yoga, pranayama, and meditation practice. For over a year I was flying high, drinking the nectar of a steady stream of insights that I felt sure would enable me to integrate the breadth and depth of SK's teachings.

At first, I was content to dig into all the individual elements of his curriculum one by one, striving to understand each on its own terms. But before too long, I began to ask myself, how do all these puzzle pieces fit together? What's the big-picture view of his spiritual path? And how can it be presented simply in a way that readers will find helpful? A second year passed with me engaged in this single-minded pursuit when my nerves began to sizzle. My inability to complete a solid first draft of the book was upsetting my equilibrium. But a reservoir of confidence remained that sooner or later my fusion of study and practice would prove potent enough to carry the day.

> *Yoga students must continually strike a balance in their contemplation of yoga's guiding principles and application of its techniques. This combination of study and practice is like a locomotive that carries an aspirant swiftly forward in their desired direction.*

A third year passed and my brain began to boil. My sleep suffered as stress-relieving dreams were replaced by circling thought-loops about the structure and content of the book. The good health I'd always enjoyed began to crumble. Yet I still had faith that providence would intervene and somehow or other my efforts would win out. When a fourth year passed without a finished product to show for it, I confided to Danna, my wife and partner on the path, one evening after dinner. "I truly don't think that I can do this. I've lost all perspective and feel like you are living with a madman obsessed." It would have been easy for Danna to retort by saying, "Tell me something I don't already know," but instead she encouraged me to keep going. Only in the wake of her kindness was I able to regain focus and do as she advised.

It's fun now to look back and make light of those five years, but their rigor was real, with me spending eight to ten hours every workday and many a weekend morning either in our yoga space or at my writing desk. Each Monday, I would enthusiastically begin anew and pour myself into a chapter only to find my writing dead ended on Friday, mirroring back my need for a more comprehensive understanding. Ouch! The truth was that something essential was lacking and I could not go forward in its absence.

I can now report that the root cause of my suffering was an erroneous blending of Swami Kripalu's renunciate and householder teachings. As all of his students knew, SK taught two paths of yoga, one for householders engaged in career and family life, and another for monks or nuns who had renounced both to practice only yoga. This was far from the first time I had confronted this dichotomy. In fact, I'd run headlong into it on the day that I met SK in 1981, while reading the opening chapter of *Science of Meditation*, which back then was his only book available in English. Eight years later and four years into our marriage, the allure of what it would be like to step beyond the limits of our householder lives was part of what drew Danna and me to quit jobs, sell a house, take monastic vows, and move into Kripalu Center as ashram residents in 1989. But hands down my hardest grapple with the topic had come in 1998, after we'd moved back to Kripalu as the dark days of the guru scandal were lifting.

> *Yoga has two paths. There is the householder path for those seeking worldly fulfillment and the renunciate path for great masters seeking liberation. The householder path is for yogis engaged in an active life in society. It builds character, bringing success and spiritual growth in equal measure. The renunciate path is for adept yogis who have abandoned worldly life and want only to free themselves from the bondage of birth and death.*

Kripalu's board of trustees had asked me to serve as president, overseeing a staff team doing the heavy lifting needed to start up a post-ashram retreat center. Alongside a myriad of operational issues, I had to reflect deeply on what the institution needed to learn from the demise of the residential ashram community, and decide how Kripalu Center's yoga curriculum should change in response. Much of this thinking occurred in 2001 at the tail end of my presidency, when I was writing *Kripalu Yoga: A Guide to Practice On and Off the Mat*.[2]

The ashram was a modern-day social experiment founded by Yogi Amrit Desai, a close student of Swami Kripalu, and built upon a reinterpretation of the age-old renunciate model. All 350 residents lived communally and took vows of poverty based on the hypothesis that its hothouse environment could metamorphose anyone willing to live the ashram lifestyle into a full-fledged monk or nun. The importance of the householder stage of life was downplayed in a push toward renunciate level practice, and the needs of individuals to discover their unique

---

[2] Kripalu Yoga is an innovative style of yoga originated by Yogi Amrit Desai and developed over several decades in collaboration with the ashram community. While inspired by and named for SK, it was never intended to replace his actual teachings.

talents, develop them to high levels, and endeavor to find success in their personal lives was largely negated.

Yogi Desai spoke directly to the ashram's renunciate orientation: "We are all such dreamers that we would like to follow the path of great masters like Swami Kripalu right away, which is the yoga of total renunciation, but this is not possible. That's why our ashram renunciation is different. The situation being created here is to bring a new dimension of growth to your life, so you can understand your mind and see for yourself how difficult it is to become a true disciple of the highest nature. We do that by taking away all the superficial stimulation, removing unhealthy food, contact with the opposite sex, distracting books and music. When you live this lifestyle, your energy begins to rise. Your magnetism increases, and the fire in your eyes becomes bright. If you can retain this energy, it will transform your life. Do not feel discouraged that you are practicing a second-rate householder yoga. Feel good that you are pursuing the highest yoga because we are combining the householder and renunciate paths in a way that enables you to grow through all the stages that lead to complete renunciation. Swami Kripalu is very clear; you have to pass through the first stage to get the second, and I am growing on this path of renunciation with you."

While in theory based on his teachings, I knew from my studies that this was never the yoga SK recommended for householders. He didn't have large ashrams in India where people came to live. Only a few swamis resided in his yoga centers, with the villagers coming and going for times of retreat and celebration. His emphasis was not enlisting renunciates but *showing householders how to weave spiritual practices into the fabric of their work and family lives.* Taking this approach, he said that a householder would progress materially and grow spiritually. If and when the calling came for deeper practice, they would be ready and able to scale the ladder of yoga to Self-realization.

Doing my best to think critically, I had to acknowledge that many residents got healthier living the ashram's lifestyle. To differing degrees, ashram life and the posture-based yoga practice it emphasized also supported their personal growth, especially during their initial years of residency. Yet it appeared to me that few ashram residents progressed all the way to a mature spiritual awakening. In the absence of a regular meditation practice and solid instruction on how to move through the advanced stages of interior contemplation, the yoga of most residents either hit a plateau or, worse yet, stagnated. The failure of this model was writ large in the married guru, who had a strong energy awakening in 1970 and afterward tried to walk the path of renunciate practice, but fell prey to outer distractions and a duplicitous life.

I thought my job was done when the Kripalu Yoga book came out in 2005 with a more householder-friendly slant, never suspecting that change of another order of magnitude was needed. And now a decade later, I was clueless that the householder/renunciate split was playing any role in my inability to complete a draft manuscript. All I knew was that my mind was circling around a vague set of contradictions and inconsistencies that it was hell-bent on resolving. Only in retrospect can I explain why my study and practice had me tiptoeing around a trap door through which I was about to fall.

MY JOURNEY DEEPENS

I was a yoga neophyte when Swami Kripalu died in 1981. Afterwards, I regarded a small cadre of his top students as my teachers. Together these unofficial successors venerated the example set by SK during his last three decades. These were the years he lived in seclusion, kept silence, and practiced ten hours a day. His earlier life in society was dismissed as time spent "exhausting his worldly karma." The most outspoken and eloquent of these students was Swami Rajarshi Muni, who minced no words in making this point: "Yoga philosophy suggests the total rejection of wealth, power, enjoyments, social affairs, economic pursuits, and all worldly activities in order to embark wholeheartedly upon a great spiritual adventure. Those who cannot turn away from society and worldly ambitions, throwing off all possessions and concerns, and breaking from all expectations and anxieties, should remain content by fixing only a modest goal for themselves on the spiritual path."[3]

Serious about my practice, I strove to embody the other-worldly ideal extolled by these senior teachers as the highest expression of yoga. This was a mindset that led me and everyone in the ashram to see the householder path as a dumbed-down derivative of the renunciate path.

---

[3] From Rajarshi Muni's book, *Yoga: The Ultimate Spiritual Path*, 116-17.

To be fair, this isn't a perspective limited to Kripalu Yoga. An ethos of renunciation pervades the yoga tradition, and Buddhism as well. But in my research, I had found a body of Swami Kripalu quotes that weren't only off this trend line—they were incompatible with this view. The best example is the pithy one that opens this book: *I encourage all my householder students, telling them: Establish yourself like a sun in the solar system of society.* Try as I may, there was no way to square this statement with a renunciate worldview. It seemed to emanate from an entirely different outlook on life.

Other quotes were more pointed, like this one explaining why different teaching models should be used to instruct householders and renunciates. Reading it, I saw a clear reference to the progressive instruction I felt was lacking in the ashram.

> *Aspirants on the householder path are taught the limbs of yoga one by one. This method of teaching is ancient and totally in accord with the experience of the rishis and sages. Through it a yogi living in society may travel fearlessly on the path of incremental progress. Grasping the eight limbs of yoga like the rungs of a ladder, a diligent householder can gradually ascend this path to samadhi. Aspirants on the renunciate path are initiated into yoga and practice all its limbs simultaneously. This method of immersion is appropriate for them, as it allows for rapid progress. But only a desireless yogi seeking liberation alone can practice the rituals of this yoga. Others find vices such as egotism, pride, and hypocrisy arising in the place of virtues.*

There were quotes that seemed to hold high the householder approach, describing its benefits as developmental prerequisites for the deeper work of spiritual awakening:

> *The regular practice of yoga is useful to both householders and renunciates. Through walking the householder path, an aspirant develops health, good character, and the following worldly powers: personal strength, determination, clear and logical thinking, good memory, creativity, and decisiveness. By learning how to direct the life energy with the mind, householders can act skillfully to fulfill their cherished*

desires while also achieving wealth, pleasure, status, and true virtue. Only after these qualities are established can the door to Self-realization be opened. Until an aspirant succeeds on the householder path, embarking on the renunciate path is like trying to jump from the earth to reach heaven.

But these were matched by other quotes that clearly placed renunciate yoga at the top of the totem pole:

Where householder yoga produces fit disciples, renunciate yoga produces great masters who have the deserving capacity to become the torch bearers of true religion and spiritual benefactors to the world. Renunciate yoga is the best yoga, as all other yogas are included in it.

In multiple places, Swami Kripalu repeated a single assertion that began to haunt my sleepless nights. I knew he was making a critical point, but somehow its full import eluded me:

Householders and renunciates follow different paths. The attention of a householder engaged in many activities is extroverted and their inner energy divided into different streams. In daily contact with the world, it can seem that innumerable thoughts and desires are created in the mind. An extroverted mind easily becomes restless and if overly agitated can shatter one's happiness to pieces. This is why householder yoga harmonizes the inner energies and aligns the mind. Not only does a householder yogi remain happy, but their unscattered mind becomes tranquil and powerful. This is what enables them to act skillfully in society, increasing their capacity to serve and attain whatever it is they desire. A renunciate withdraws from the world to escape the bondage of mind. In renunciate yoga, the life energy is allowed to surge powerfully through the system. This dissolves the bonds of mental impressions but also renders the mind unstable. Self-control can be lost at any time in response to an unexpected stimulation. This is why a renunciate yogi must live in seclusion. These paths are completely different. Each has its own scriptures and scriptural interpretations, so it is not fruitful to compare them.

His unequivocal statement that *these paths are completely different* flew in the face of the idea that householder yoga was a derivative of anything else. But as a student, I had never been taught the householder path in an affirmative fashion, one that respected its distinctive tenets and spoke to its highest possibilities. Much to the contrary, I practiced yoga as a renunciate wannabe. This mismatch of my householder life with a monkish mindset caused me considerable distress. It left me dogged by a feeling that there was a higher path than the one I was following. Instead of helping me channel the energy generated by my practice into my work and marriage, it was an archetype at odds with my actual circumstances. And now, in writing a guide for other practitioners, I intuitively sensed that the blending of these paths was not a superficial blemish in the teachings I'd received. It was a tectonic fault hidden at their core. While long overdue in my obligation to produce a draft manuscript, I knew on some level that it was not right to pass on this faulty householder meme. Stuck on the horns of this dilemma, I was in crisis.

Revelation came to my rescue by way of serendipity. In despair, I shifted my focus back to Swami Kripalu's biography. I'd long ago drafted a life sketch and returned there to review it and avoid the pain of all my other failures. It was in the midst of reworking the story of his early life that my epiphany began to unfold. Its opening salvo reminded me of this line drawing of a duck, gazing right over its open bill.

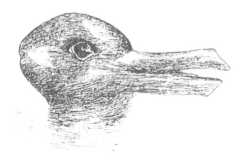

Looking again, can you see the rabbit looking to the left with its ears pointing right? This is what psychologists call an ambiguous image. It's both a duck and a rabbit, but once your brain has interpreted the drawing one way it's difficult to see the other, and almost impossible to see both of them simultaneously. One afternoon, while straining my eyes to read a faded lecture transcript, a novel question arose in my mind: What if SK's teachings are this kind of amalgam?

At this point, I only knew Swami Kripalu as an ardent monk. Moreover, I'd been inoculated with a view that habituated me to seeing only his renunciate yoga. Metaphorically speaking, I was fixated on the duck and blind to the rabbit. In focusing on his life story prior to becoming a swami, I began to see the householder path that he'd actually walked into midlife, when he was an ambitious young man endeavoring to support his widowed mother and make his way in the world. Closely tracking through this formative period, it became obvious where all the elements of his householder yoga had originated. I could also see how its practice had carried him into a decade of being what I came to call "a self-actualizing swami." These were significant years during which he became a celebrated orator and humanitarian, inspiring good works on a regional scale that eventually led to his national recognition.

It was important for me to discover that Swami Kripalu had not set aside his drives and desires to pursue a renunciate ideal. Much to the contrary, it was these passions that fueled his ardor for self-development. When fulfilled, they led seamlessly to his energetic awakening and the single-minded yoga practice that he performed afterward in seclusion. Contemplating his life in this fashion, I was not only able to glimpse the rabbit of his householder yoga but pull it out of the hat and examine it closely. I was incredulous. For all these years, I'd only been seeing half the picture. And more importantly, the whole Kripalu Center organization had made a similar mistake.

Epiphany followed on the heels of this life review, a moment in morning meditation when a clear knowing dawned that was striking only in its simplicity. It illumined each element of the householder path and left me feeling that I had grasped the essence of what SK sometimes called *the yoga of engagement*.[4] Gone was the dry asceticism so long at the center of my yoga practice. In its place was a juicy aliveness that was emotionally buoyant. Then I watched as a turn of mind took place that produced a virtual mirror-image of the renunciate worldview. Human embodiment is not a soul-trap or shackle to escape, but an opportunity to bring spirit into form by consciously infusing all our actions with its vital energy, and

---

[4] Later I found that SK categorized this experience as *yoga darshana* in which a practitioner receives a clear vision of their rightful path and where it is leading—see chapter 9. The opposite of the householder *yoga of engagement* is the renunciate *yoga of cessation* in which a practitioner seeks to dissolve the mind and identify exclusively with the unborn and deathless.

embracing challenges as invitations for growth. As this alternative mindset took shape, I realized that to the extent I'd walked this life-affirming path I had met with success. And whenever I'd wandered off it, some degree of difficulty had ensued. For the first time, I was a happy householder.

I returned to my studies with new eyes and was surprised to find this positive view winking back at me from all four corners of SK's teachings. In places, its key elements were expressly stated. More often, it was encoded in shorthand references to a doctrine called *the four aims of life*,[5] and symbolically conveyed in the stories he told. There were holes and missing pieces—places where I've needed to connect the dots—but never for a moment did it seem that I was inventing something new. This was his vision of yoga for people living active lives, and my first task was to bring it alive in myself. In the five years since that seismic shift, I've worked to articulate this life-hardy mindset by culling a treasure trove of SK quotes to inform the practice of householder yogis and coupling them with a narrative storyline and commentary.

The yoga of engagement teaches us to enjoy our journey through life. First it shows us how to attend to the health of body and mind, as these vehicles must be made to work effectively to undertake the journey. Then it brings forth all our positive capacities, many of which have been with us since childhood, to ensure our success. To complete the journey, many spiritual qualities are also necessary. If

---

[5] Yoga recognizes four noble aims of life: dharma or right living, artha or material security, kama or enjoyment, and moksha or spiritual liberation—see chapter 5. Where householders pursue a balance of all four, renunciates pursue only the last. SK taught that renunciation was appropriate for select aspirants called to withdraw from society and *practice yoga and only yoga for the rest of their lives*. It's easy to see how a renunciate mindset could serve cloistered monks and nuns by reinforcing their chosen vocation and motivating them to focus exclusively on their spiritual practice. There may also be a stage in human development, or a time in the life cycle, where a turning away from the things of this world is healthy for non-monks as well. I am not attacking renunciation per se, but simply agreeing with what SK taught: a renunciate outlook on life is not well-suited to the needs of most yoga students, including many individuals highly motivated to progress in their practice. This book may ruffle the feathers of those accustomed to seeing his teachings through a strictly renunciate lens, as in places I will be describing something they've always seen as a duck's hard and pointy bill as the soft and furry ears of a rabbit. I ask those readers to remember that my intention is not to undermine the renunciate view. I am simply presenting an alternate perspective that my research and life experience suggests has equal legitimacy.

> *we try to obtain these all at once, we invariably fail, so yoga brings them into being one by one. This is why I can confidently say that a householder yogi intent on making this journey will succeed in their worldly life and progress spiritually too.*

By far the most egregious error in the ashram teachings I received was a presumption that the householder path cannot lead an aspirant all the way to Self-realization (atman darshan), a stage that many contemporary teachers equate with the end point of the spiritual path. Both my study and practice leave me certain this presumed limitation is untrue. Swami Kripalu's householder yoga aims to carry aspirants to and across this auspicious threshold, after which they have everything required to enjoy a vibrant and evolving inner life, while maintaining a dynamic outer life as well. Yet he did not conflate Self-realization and the high levels of human fulfillment it makes possible with yoga's ultimate goal, which is nothing short of the complete emancipation of the soul. As SK demonstrated in his own life, Self-realization is not a final attainment but a prerequisite for liberation.

> *As direct knowledge dawns, doubts recede as the screen of illusion covering the intellect is removed and Self-realization is attained. Lord Krishna in the Bhagavad Gita calls a Self-realized yogi "one who is self-possessed" and explains why this beyond-mind state must be seen and stabilized to control the senses and overcome bodily identification. Maharishi Patanjali in his Yoga Sutra teaches that with Self-realization faith is greatly enhanced, and the polarities of pain and pleasure no longer distract. It is only after crossing to this stage that a yogi's inner journey will not be cut short by various obstacles. Such a yogi is able to gain health, nobility, respect, wealth, and other accomplishments. But only one who continues the path all the way to liberation is a complete yogi.*

Bringing my view, practice, and direct experience into alignment has made the power of yoga available to me. I know that for me, life is not a zero-sum game in which the things of this world must be given up to know God. It's a precious opportunity for a soul-seed to grow into a fully-expressed human being and blossom spiritually in the light of Self-realization. Just as Swami Kripalu taught and modeled, the best way to foster this growth is not to withdraw into seclusion but step forward to claim our *dharma*, or life calling. Then we can act purposefully to heal our wounds and traumas, bring forth budding capacities, learn how to discharge our duties joyfully, hone the skills needed to maximize our contribution to society, and realize the presence of spirit in the midst of an engaged life. If the householder path has a credo, it might be that you have to make your way in the world to know God. Yoga practice is a tremendous ally in this process, and a healthy mix of discipline and discernment is certainly required, but self-denial and an ascetic disavowal of daily life is not.

Insights, epiphanies, and breakthroughs of all kinds are traveling companions on the path of yoga. The traditional guidance is not to make much of them. Yet I felt this one was worth recounting because of the pivotal role it played in the genesis of this book. When illustrative, other personal anecdotes and incidents from Kripalu Center's ashram past appear in the chapters that follow.[6] In a lifetime of study and practice, I have found no better approach to yoga than the one I discovered hiding in plain sight in Swami Kripalu's householder teachings.[7] May it prove as valuable to you as it has been for me.

---

[6] The yoga tradition advises students to only share personal experiences with their guru, or other students of their guru doing the same practices, to avoid the risk of self-aggrandizement. Yet by far the most helpful books I've found have been ones in which the authors were straightforward and self-disclosing. Because this book is likely to have an audience with a Kripalu Center connection, I have opted to treat its readers as what the yoga tradition would consider brother and sister yoga students.

[7] Every system seeking to guide a student's growth and development has shortcomings and problem areas. At the end of the final book in this series, I offer some critiques but they are only worthy of consideration after a thorough presentation of SK's approach.

PART TWO
GRASP THE ESSENCE OF YOGA

Here is the guidance of the supremely kind and knowledgeable truth teachers of the past. First grasp the essence of yoga. Then abandon all concerns and enthusiastically engage yourself in its practice.

Swami Kripalu was a renowned yogi who lived in seclusion and rarely taught publicly. All the speeches he delivered in India were special events attended by crowds that numbered in the thousands. Even in America, where he actively shunned the spotlight, his discourses always drew a sizeable group of dedicated students, a small retinue of Indian swamis, and a smattering of people new to yoga. In addressing these mixed audiences, he was careful to provide something of interest to everyone.

The chief purpose of all my talks—past, present, and future—is to inspire you in practical ways that can enhance your life. Today I have tried to remain vigilant so each of you can receive the guidance you desire regardless of whether you're a beginner, intermediate, or advanced student. Every word of this discourse is filled with my experience of yoga sadhana (ardent practice) and scripture study. If you read and reflect on it regularly, you will gain new insights and realizations, as the teachings are understood differently in different stages of practice.

SK was a gifted orator able to braid these disparate strands into captivating lectures that edified his diverse listeners. However, the library of transcribed talks left behind for me to study was a hodgepodge of teachings. I turned my attention to his major written works hoping to discover an overview of yoga to orient my practice, but I found them difficult and in places cryptic.[1] That led me to search for a translated version of the entry-level instruction he must have given new students in India. I failed to locate anything comprehensive, only more nuggets of pertinent advice scattered here and there throughout his talks and writings. It just wasn't easy to sort out his guidance to a novice English-speaking practitioner like myself, which made it frustrating to encounter statements emphasizing the importance of yoga's fundamentals.

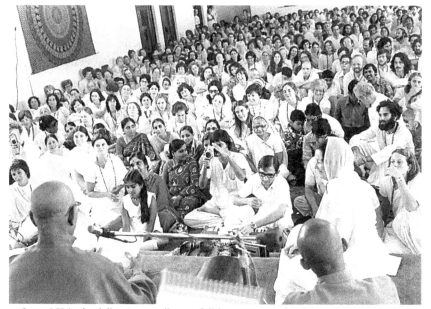

Swami Kripalu delivering a talk to a full house soon after his arrival in America.

Yoga provides a set of principles that form a foundation for practice. Your first step as a student should be to learn those principles. By gaining this knowledge, you will develop a strong conviction in the yogic approach. Practice should not begin before this approach is understood, as all students are bound to encounter difficulties. Where students with guiding principles display a purposefulness that enables them to generate enthusiasm and overcome obstacles,

---

[1] Only later did I learn that key portions of SK's major works were written in a symbolic form of expression called sandha-bhasa (twilight language) used to safeguard the secrets of kundalini yoga. This is what made sections of them appear cryptic.

those that start prematurely become confused and cannot stick to the path. This is not their fault; it is the result of a wavering mind that never understood the first principles.

While doing this detective work, I kept running into places where SK stressed the value of *systematic practice*. At first, I thought he meant doing the poses in the right order. Later I imagined that he was talking about properly combining postures with other techniques such as yogic breathing, conscious relaxation, and sitting meditation. Only gradually did it dawn on me that I was engaged in what he called *haphazard practice*. While faithful in my routines, I was pretty much clueless about what I was trying to accomplish by doing them.

Most people do yoga without understanding the principles, objectives, and secrets of its techniques. This haphazard practice is a lot like the punishment meted out fifty years ago in Indian primary schools, where teachers made errant students bend down, touch their toes, and remain in this position. This is the hands-to-feet pose, which aids digestion by massaging the abdomen and sharpens the intellect by supplying blood to the brain. No form of practice ever goes to waste, and even a person doing postures in a mechanical fashion receives benefits. But a knowledgeable student practicing yoga systematically experiences rapid progress. Within a short time, they begin to undergo pleasant and mysterious experiences. Enjoying these benefits, they become extremely interested in yoga and their faith in its efficacy increases day by day. An industrious student like this, if given proper guidance, will progress into the advanced stages of yoga.

When Swami Kripalu was nineteen years old, he met a guru who adopted him as a spiritual son and spent the next fifteen months schooling him in the precepts of yoga. As a new practitioner, I felt this same need, wanting someone older and wiser to put their hand on my shoulder and point the way forward. More than technical on-the-mat instruction, I needed to understand how yoga's guiding principles and practices fit together to form a coherent approach to life. Having scoured everything at my disposal and come up empty, all I could do was return to the mixed bag of teachings before me and try to compile a primer for myself. Steeping myself in these materials, it was obvious that SK's teachings arose from an organizing vision of yoga, but there were missing pieces that kept me from understanding and practicing in the purposeful way he suggested was possible.

> *A practitioner ignorant of yoga's essence is like a person wandering around in the pitch dark. Gaining the light of this knowledge is the first imperative, as with it everything else in the spiritual life can be accomplished. Progress in yoga requires the clear sense of direction born from a doubt-free knowledge of its path. A person deviating right and left cannot carry out its pilgrimage. When the essence of yoga is grasped, knowledge and confidence unite, energy ignites, and systematic practice ensues.*

Eventually I stumbled on an anomaly that proved an important clue. In a series of discourses delivered in America, SK described yoga as the search for happiness. This stood out from the majority of his Indian teachings, where yoga was viewed as the practice of austerities performed to transcend the limits of body and mind, bringing religious revelation and bestowing extraordinary powers. Reading these American discourses carefully, I could see that he was characterizing yoga as a pathway to a rich and rewarding life. Instead of adopting an ascetic mindset, its practices could be done to nurture the body, fine tune the mind, and bring high levels of human development into reach. Looking back, I can say that I'd found a basic tenet of the householder path, and a view of yoga that would have currency with today's practitioners. At the time, I only knew that SK was intellectually rigorous and this new depiction of yoga no casual mistake.

> *The nature of the human mind is to roam everywhere in search of happiness. As long as our search is focused externally, the mind will be unduly influenced by circumstances and experiences outside of its control. Growing more and more agitated, such a mind tends to become miserable, and it can seem that one's hope for happiness is in vain. Yet this great ocean of unhappiness can be crossed. First become a philosopher by sitting calmly and thinking clearly about*

the path before you in life. Next become a scientist by testing your ideas. Adjust your habits to foster the health of the body. Attend to your duties with enthusiasm and concentration. Watch to see if your maturing practice pacifies the mind, bringing it more under your control and making your actions effective. Then one fine day become a yogi by entering the root of your being and discovering the complete knowledge and peace that lies unsuspected there. Everything entailed in this process of harmonizing the body and mind and eventually going beyond the limitations of both is yoga, the trustworthy means of attaining a lasting happiness.

I was certain that SK knew Western thinking was rooted in the philosophy of the ancient Greeks, who believed that all human beings strive for eudemonia, a state of well-being and flourishing. This motivated me to revisit their writings, where I found a few ideas common to eastern and western classical thought that patched the holes in my understanding of his householder yoga. It's easy for anyone exposed to renunciate ideals to imagine that a yoga practitioner's search for mundane happiness simply gets replaced by a quest for an other-worldly enlightenment. On the path SK walked and taught, the search for worldly happiness grows into a passion for growth that brings self-actualization and outer success. Then, by enabling depth interior practice, it culminates in Self-realization.[2]

Were you to visit me in India, you would find that my library has books on all the world's religions and spiritual traditions. From early childhood, I have studied these books with great love, not to become a philosopher but simply to understand the truth in them. I am interested in the religion that holds high the divine potential

---

[2] Self-actualization is a psychological term that describes a developmental process in which one's latent potentials are brought into expression or "actualized." It was introduced in the early half of the twentieth by Kurt Goldstein, a physician specializing in neuroanatomy and psychiatry. Self-realization is a term that appears to have originated around the same time, both in the East/West psychology of Carl Jung and in the interface of Eastern gurus including Paramahansa Yogananda and Western yoga students. Self-realization is technically not the result of any process. It is regaining awareness and knowledge of one's true nature, which for a time was lost to consciousness. Thanks to friend and Kripalu Center board member, Steve Dinkelaker, for pointing me back to the teachings of the ancient Greek sages.

of every individual, the religion that includes everyone and doesn't exclude anyone by unduly praising any particular country, culture, or sect. While I've found this in yoga, all the world's sages and scriptures testify to this selfsame truth.

The next few chapters trace the journey I made to assemble Swami Kripalu's introductory teachings into a coherent narrative. I hope it enables you to engage in the type of informed practice he valued without wasting as much time as I did bush-whacking in the dark.

CHAPTER 3
GIFT OF THE SAGES

India is the land of the rishis and sages who lived in the forest and practiced strict austerities for thousands of years to develop the science of yoga. The spiritual principles discovered by these early yogis are not ordinary. They are extraordinary and enable an aspirant to step beyond the limits of body and mind to enter the otherwise unapproachable realm of the soul.

Swami Kripalu held the sages of ancient India in high esteem and considered yoga their gift to the world. Proud of his cultural heritage, he might have sat down with a brand-new student and delivered the following "history lesson" to shed light on the origins of this holistic approach to self-development and spiritual awakening now practiced by millions around the globe.

* * *

The roots of yoga reach back to the visionary *rishis* or "seers" who founded Indian culture. The rishis intuitively sensed the presence of an inner unity underlying the diversity of the natural world. They named it *Brahman*, the Absolute, and sang its praises in the oral canon of religious hymns, mystical poetry, and ritualistic incantations that centuries later would become the written Vedas.[1] The rishis envisioned Brahman as the

---

[1] The word *veda* means knowledge and is a derivative of the root vid which means to know. The four Vedas are the seminal Indian scriptures. Composed around 3000 BCE, they are the oldest books in humankind's library. The word yoga appears in the Vedas and has multiple meanings. In places, it is likened to a chariot that enables a long journey to be safely and expeditiously completed, a definition that meshes well with SK's approach.

singular power from which the cosmos emerged, a supreme principle that was the cause of everything, including their gods. All the visible forces of nature were seen to have their source in this invisible ground of being, and the rishis imagined that anyone gaining access to Brahman would discover an inexhaustible reservoir of energy and intelligence lying at the heart of creation. Their highest aspiration was to find a way to harness this hidden power so individuals could actualize their potential and society could not just survive but flourish.

Inspired by the rishis' vision, generations of men and women renounced conventional life to dedicate themselves whole-heartedly to the search for Brahman. Banding together in forest hermitages, isolating themselves in remote mountain caves, and dwelling on the fringes of the urban centers that sprang up along the Indus and later Ganges rivers, they lived as ascetic sages. The word yoga is derived from the root *yuj*, which means "to join or yoke," and these sages experimented with a broad spectrum of techniques to bind their individual soul to the cosmic soul of Brahman.

Some sages tried to unlock the secret of Brahman by winning the favor of the gods. Striving to be virtuous and worthy of boons, they developed a system of ritual sacrifice called yajna. Others undertook rigorous disciplines to gain paranormal powers and bring the ungraspable Brahman into reach. They developed the practice of austerities known as tapas. Some sages sharpened their intellects to discern if there was a hierarchy hidden in the fabric of creation that could be used to mentally ascend from the material world to Brahman. They developed a metaphysical taxonomy distinguishing spirit from matter called Samkhya. Other sages explored the life-giving breath believed to arise from Brahman. They developed the techniques of breath regulation called pranayama. Still others fixated their attention to stop the mind and see if Brahman lies beyond thought. They developed the art of meditation called dhyana. With iron-willed endurance, all these sages sought contact with an ultimate reality they conceived as other than themselves.

The great sages of ancient times abandoned the comforts of society to establish yoga. The yoga they practiced was not just meditation. Meditation was combined with many physical and intellectual activities. They purged themselves of vices, filling the void thus created with virtues. They faced reality and found out how the mind works. Eventually they discovered the source of the body and mind where the soul becomes one with the Supreme Spirit.

Useful knowledge was gained from all these pursuits, but trial and error eventually led these innovative sages to move away from any outer-directed avenues of seeking. Turning their attention inward, the sages drew elements from each of these approaches to piece together an introspective path to Brahman. Its initial stages were crafted to optimize the functioning of body and mind. Its end stages were focused on attaining direct spiritual knowledge. Pioneering this path, some sages rose to high levels of illumination. Communities formed around them, and their teachings were recorded in a remarkable set of texts called the Upanishads.[2] Old texts were circulated and new ones written as the tenets of yoga took shape in the creative interplay of these insightful sages.

The ancient rishis approached yoga scientifically with this firm conviction: If one person has attained the highest consciousness, then others can too. If there was one great master, there can be another by applying the same principles and practices. In today's world, a person studies postures and becomes a yoga teacher a short time later. The sages who wrote the Upanishads only did so after a thousand years of collective study and experimentation. These texts are a vast storehouse of yogic experience. No matter what type of yoga you choose to pursue, you will see your questions addressed and answered in them.

Together the Upanishadic sages made a ground-breaking discovery. The vision of the rishis was prophetic and true. Both our individual bodies and the vast and ever-changing world we perceive with our mind and

---

[2] *Upanishad* means *to sit at the feet of a master* and these texts record the spiritual dialogues of sages living as forest hermits with their close disciples. Almost two hundred Upanishads were written between the seventh and first century BCE. Their content varies widely and includes philosophical speculation, spiritual teaching, yoga instruction, and archaic religious lore. Some scholars consider the Bhagavad Gita a crowning Upanishad because it was written at the end of this era and distils their teachings into a cogent yoga-based approach to living. Many later texts were written that call themselves "Upanishads," including an influential set of "Yoga Upanishads," but these should be understood as coming from a different historical period.

senses emerges from an unchanging inner core of being, which radiates a life-giving energy that can be used for good. Super-human abilities are not required to access this interior dimension of reality; it is more a matter of looking in the right place. In the words of the Upanishads, the transcendent Brahman is elusive and hard to find anywhere in creation, but it can be realized through the immanent and indwelling *atman*, a word simply meaning "self."

> *You can't find the seed from which a great tree sprouted in its roots, trunk, or countless branches. You have to look inside the fruit. The same is true with Brahman. Even though it is the source of everything, Brahman cannot be found anywhere externally. You have to look inside yourself to find the hidden seed of atman. And that seed in you has the same power that formed the universe.*

Atman is not the surface ego, a deeper layer of the psyche, or an exalted mind state. All of these were well-known to the ancient sages. The doorway to Brahman that answered their quest was something qualitatively different. They experienced atman as metaphysical—beyond matter—a spark of pure energy and free awareness existing on a dimension entirely off the map of normal perception.

Instead of a thing or object, atman is better understood as our source point for the inflow of life energy that inspires the breath, animates the body, illumines the mind, and enlivens the senses. This energy plays a central role in yoga. Some Upanishads refer to it as *atman shakti*, the power of the self. Swami Kripalu preferred a simpler term used in other Upanishads that appears often in this book: *prana*, the life force. Atman is also our access point to the all-pervading field of pure consciousness that links us to Brahman, an unsuspected portal or wormhole beyond the limits of body and mind that makes yoga's ultimate goals of Self-realization and spiritual liberation possible.

All of yoga is best understood as a process of forging a direct connection to this energetic core of our being, opening to its transformative power, aligning with its creative intelligence, enjoying the sense of peace and expansiveness it bestows, and channeling its outpouring energy into our lives. All of yoga's teachings and techniques are meant to serve this overarching goal. Truly, it is a practitioner's intention to use the tools of postures, pranayama, and meditation to tap into this wellspring of vital energy and bring forth the full power of the self that makes something yoga.

Yoga has only one goal, union with Brahman, but it can be reached through various pathways as detailed in the Upanishads. Whatever type of yoga one practices, its aim should be atman-darshan (direct self-knowing). Then only does the term yoga apply.

The reason why the Upanishadic sages' discovery of atman was—and remains—an epic breakthrough is because it was not uttered as religious doctrine or philosophy. The sages developed yoga as a rigorous wisdom tradition with techniques that can be applied by anyone to validate or disprove its assertions in the laboratory of their own body-mind. The practice of yogic techniques is an indispensable part of the experiment, as layers of distraction and mental conditioning must be cut through before the extroverted awareness flowing out through the senses can be turned back to realize its source in atman and Brahman.

The ancient rishis sought a supreme knowledge that proved extremely difficult to obtain. This knowledge of Brahman cannot be found in the Vedas, Upanishads, or any other books. You have to descend into the body, enter into consciousness, and get close to the soul. This is the only way to receive this absolute knowledge. When the sages discovered atman, they found that we all have tremendous power, but only if we connect ourselves with Brahman, like train cars coupled to a locomotive. Yoga is the science they developed that enables you to connect to Brahman with ease.

WHAT MAKES A WISDOM TRADITION?

Yoga is one of the world's oldest wisdom traditions boldly proclaiming that life-transforming truth exists and humans have the capacity to know it directly. All wisdom traditions are composed of three building blocks: a view, a practice, and the direct experience of the practitioner.

- A view (darshana) is a particular way of seeing yourself and the world around you. A good view provides you

with a solid intellectual framework to inform your practice and a clear map to guide your journey to truth. A good view also has conceptual models designed to help you navigate known obstacles and pitfalls.
- Practice (abhyasa) gives you a method to inquire deeply into the nature of reality and test the validity of the view. An effective practice activates the life force of the body, heightens self-awareness, awakens intuition, and grants access to deeper states of consciousness.
- Direct experience (anubhava) is the first-hand knowledge that comes from the unmediated contact with reality made possible by focused practice. By drinking again and again from the fount of direct experience, your view will evolve to encompass more of life's mysteries.

The view of a wisdom tradition is qualitatively different than religion, philosophy, an ideology, or even a system of metaphysics, because it's not adopted as ultimate truth. A wisdom tradition puts forth a view as a working hypothesis to be validated or discarded in the experimental fire of practice. It is understood from the beginning that direct experience will evolve and eventually shatter the view to replace it with revelatory truth. A wisdom tradition is not meant to enlist followers; it empowers you to explore and find out for yourself. Throughout this book, a variety of different views and models embraced by SK will be presented. It's your job as a reader to determine which of them you want to explore through practice.

Looking at the lives of the great rishis and sages leads to the conclusion that the higher stages of yoga are not accessible through logic or reason; they are accessible only through direct experience.

BE A DISCERNING STUDENT

Swami Kripalu's view of Indian history tracked with everything I'd read in my undergraduate studies of world religions. It added a yoga practitioner's perspective that I found helpful and inspiring. It even included an explanation of how the householder and renunciate paths arose early in yoga's development, which in my mind cemented his belief in their distinctness:

> *In the forests of ancient India, many saints and sages lived and died with yoga as their goal in life. In those days, renunciation was not an attitude donned by all. Some sages were single ascetics. Others were married couples, partners in the holy life who shared a love for yoga. These two groups lived in their own ways, carrying out their practices with great enthusiasm. The people living in the surrounding towns and villages were highly impressed by these forest dwelling sages. They considered them apta purushas, trustworthy souls who had experienced the Absolute (Brahman) and spoke only truth. They studied the texts written by these sages and adopted the same ideals. Benefitting from the support of the people, the sages strove to develop ways to share what they had discovered and learned with them. It was in those days, when saints were predominant and purity prevailed in the minds of the common people, that the two paths of yoga emerged.*

In the four decades since his death, yoga's popularity has generated considerable academic interest. Today's scholars would consider his account of the rishis a romanticized tale of yoga's origins. Instead of enlightened seers, the historical record depicts the founders of Indian culture as nomadic cattle herders with a strong warrior ethic and passion for sacred hymns and ecstatic poetry. While the word Brahman appears in the Vedas, it is only vaguely defined and used in contradictory ways. Its characterization as the Absolute ground of being only appears much later in the Upanishads.

More importantly, it's become clear that yoga's true history is highly nuanced and the task of reconstructing it exceptionally complex. Instead of a single system that developed early and remained consistent over time, yoga-like practices were integral to a multiplicity of early Indian religious sects with widely-diverging doctrines. Like all sophisticated fields of knowledge, yoga evolved over a considerable span of time. A good argument can be made that it did not become an integrated approach until 1000 CE. Even more surprising, much of what we associate with yoga arose in the early twentieth century when indigenous views and practices were blended with Western elements in a modernizing makeover that produced the transnational posture-based practice so popular today.

Swami Kripalu was clearly not alone in holding the rose-colored vision of the rishis schooled into him in the 1930s. It became the prevailing historical narrative in the mid-to-late 1800s when it was put forth by the leaders of India's independence movement to restore pride in their country's spiritual heritage. Their goal was to create the national identity needed to oppose British colonialism. Over the next century and a half, a long line of eminent western Orientalists from Max Müller (1823-1900) to Georg Feuerstein (1947-2012) echoed this idealized view. So did the procession of Indian gurus who brought yoga to America that started with Swami Vivekananda in 1894 and reached its peak in the 1960s and 70s.

As a student of yoga, I've come to accept that the scholars are undoubtedly correct in the domain of history. I think SK would want me to point out his outdated historical view, as he encouraged all his students to be independent thinkers.

I never take anything for granted simply because it appears in a text or is said by an expert. I always test it myself and will only accept something as truth after it is confirmed by my own experience. Even in a simple matter like doing the headstand, ten experts will give you ten different opinions on how to do so correctly. Only after analyzing their advice and conducting your own experiments can you arrive at the one answer you need to progress in your practice.

The Upanishadic sages knew this principle. When one of them reached a climax in meditation, the others did not immediately accept it as final and say, "This is the highest realization and all the truth that can be experienced." Instead, they closely observed and reflected upon it. Often, they found it was only the end of one stage and entry into the next. That is how yoga progressed further and further.

It is necessary for all of us to learn the fundamentals of yoga from others. But after that you must make a special effort to digest each and every principle. First exercise your logic and reasoning ability. Then engage in your own experiments to test whether a teaching is correct. By practicing in this way, the power of your discrimination will increase until your mentality is operating on a high level. As direct knowing dawns, more and more truth will become visible to you.

Despite these differences in opinion, today's scholars would agree with SK that yoga-like practices date back to the dawn of Indian civilization and the tradition took shape over millennia through the painstaking efforts of its countless sages.

APPLYING THIS CHAPTER IN PRACTICE

While not factual, SK's tale of the rishis is a meaningful myth that points out a clear North Star that can lead you forward in your practice. The essence of yoga is not a posture, a breathing exercise, or a state of meditation. It's following the example of yoga's founding sages by using these and other disciplines to access the universal power and intelligence lying dormant within you through the doorway of the inner self. Contemporary posture-based yoga is criticized for having lost its spirit, but what this means is often equated with a disregard for the niceties of Indian culture. Yoga's true spirituality arises not from its outer trappings, but from its ability to reveal your inner incandescence. Oriented to this guiding intention to tap into the power of your own energetic source, you can effectively engage the various tools and teachings of yoga to revitalize the body, illumine the mind, and actualize your potentials in all areas of life.

I remember my introduction to the term atman, and a little later, Buddha-nature, in a comparative religion class. At the time, I was a junior in college struggling to make my way in life through a mental maze of opposites and running headlong into all sorts of push/pull conflicts. My inner state meshed with what I'd learned in Psychology 101, where the thankless role of the self or ego is to mediate between the instinctual drives of the assertive id and the restraining ideals of the superego. With the conscious mind likened to the visible tip of an iceberg, and the majority of our behavior said to be driven by more powerful forces submerged in the subconscious and unconscious, all my efforts to grow and change felt like losing propositions.[3]

Inwardly divided and plagued by uncertainty, I wanted to believe that my being was grounded in something deeper than my right/wrong thinking mind. It was appealing to imagine the unconscious as a repository of spiritual knowledge able to resolve life's mysteries, among the deepest of which is the nature of consciousness itself. But those Eastern ideas alone did little to shift my experience of inner mud wrestling. Several years would have to pass before I met SK and found a way to test the truth of yoga's radical assertion that everyone has an umbilical-like connection to the whole of everything that is potent enough to overcome the deficits of the polarizing thinking mind.

In ancient India, a new student was carefully taught the principles of yoga before undertaking any practice. These principles were called siddhanta, a compound word with a clear meaning. A siddha is a great yogi who accomplished samadhi and realized the ultimate truth. The syllable "anta" means "established principle." Thus, the siddhantas are the established principles of yoga that contain the seed experience of the great sages. There are two founding principles: (1) Brahman is the source and cause of the whole universe; and (2) Brahman can be known directly through atman, which brings fresh energy into the system and enables one to grow spiritually and end suffering. But to attain Brahman and make wise use of its energy, one must commence a consistent yoga practice while continuing to contemplate all the other siddhantas.

---

[3] This psychological view of the self reflects the psychoanalytic theory of Sigmund Freud, who was the first to propose the iceberg metaphor of the conscious, subconscious, and unconscious minds that is still in use today. At the time, I wasn't aware of Freud's protege Carl Jung, who saw the ego as the outward-facing mask of a deeper self that encompasses the entirety of the iceberg. In Jung's analytical psychology, the self is connected to a "collective unconscious" that is shared by humankind as a whole. In Jungian therapy, the collective unconscious is considered the source of archetypal energies and intuitive wisdom able to catalyze rapid psychological and spiritual growth in a process called individuation. Many contemporary psychologies envision the self in ways compatible with yoga.

CHAPTER 4
EMPOWERMENT THROUGH SELF-DISCOVERY

Dear aspirant! If yoga is done without first knowing the atman underlying the activity of the mind and senses, it is lifeless and soulless. In this state, real progress is impossible. Consider your body pulsing with energy as a laboratory to enter and practice yoga. Then take atman as your teacher.

Even as a novice yogi, I could tell that Swami Kripalu was not spouting philosophy when he directed students to look inside themselves to find the hidden seed of atman. He was pointing to a reality outside the scope of our normal awareness. Atman was not a metaphysical abstraction to him. It was real and palpable, the energetic source of our aliveness, and something you can experience right now.

Close your eyes and bring your attention inside. Draw in a long inhalation and let out a relaxing sigh. Now find the point at the center of the mind and senses by asking yourself, "Who is it that sees, hears, smells, tastes, and feels?" If focusing your awareness in this way seems awkward, or even a bit uncomfortable, stick with the inquiry. Don't be surprised if you find this center point more verb than noun, a radiating spark of inner aliveness.

There is a name for this place at the confluence of all five senses—the sensorium—and the yogis considered it a doorway (*dwara*) between the inner and outer worlds. As your attention steadies, you are likely to discover that this center point is both static and dynamic, a stillness that pulsates with life energy. Although it can be likened to a point, closer inspection will reveal that this is not completely accurate. It is a focal point without a center, a dot of awareness whose physical location can't be pinned down because it exists on a different and deeper dimension of reality.

If your focus grows strong, you may find this tiny point expanding into a vast field of awareness or all-pervading presence. The Svetasvatara Upanishad graphically describes this paradox of scale in verse 5.9, "This living atman is to be known as a part within, smaller than one hundredth the tip of a hair, subdivided once again a hundredfold, and yet it partakes of infinity."

Our minds are restless. This restlessness is caused by the contact of our five senses with the outside world. To steady our mind, we must make it introvert by closing the gates of our senses to outside stimulation. By cutting off this external stimulation, even for a short time, we can go within and attune to the life energy that emanates from atman.

Keeping the eyes closed, shift your attention to sense whatever is changing in the environment around you. This is likely to include sounds, smells, and the movement of air on your skin, which the yogis described as being experienced through the "sense gates" connecting you to the world outside. Then bring your attention back inside and notice any feelings, thoughts, or images flowing internally through the mechanism of the mind, which assembles the input of the senses into the outer world we experience, and stores select impressions as memory.[1] Now return to the still point at the center of all motion, the core of your identity that enables you to register all these things through the vehicle of the mind and senses.

As you master the art of entering within, you will get more energy. The deeper the roots of the tree, the more sustenance it can draw

---

[1] The ancient yogis considered the mind a sixth sense because it operates from a database of past sense impressions retained in memory. Today the term sixth sense is used by people who believe that humans have extrasensory abilities. The yogis agree that the human mind has a range of extrasensory capacities, which can be cultivated through persistent practice. But before such practice can bear fruit, the thinking mind that we experience day-in and day-out must be understood as sense-based and limited, which opens the door to depth meditation.

into itself. When you can draw close to the soul, you will obtain the power and purity of atman.

Yoga teaches that hidden at the root of our capacity to sense whatever is changing around or within us is something constant and unchanging. This changeless element is atman, our true self and spiritual source. While easy to overlook, it's from this still point that life force infuses the body and the impetus to breathe originates.[2] It's from here that energy enlivens the senses and awareness illumines the mind. It's from here that out-of-the-box creativity springs forth, intuitive knowing emerges, and love kindles its glow in the heart. This is our power point, the place from which we can make conscious choices and exercise our agency to act. Simply by focusing our awareness on this source point, the inner doorway to atman opens a little wider, and its life-giving energy streams into our being to revitalize and quicken us.

Once someone asked me, "What is atman?" and I responded, "Have you seen a living person? Have you seen a dead body? The difference between these two is atman." Atman is the principle of aliveness. Everyone believes they perform actions through the medium of the body, mind, and ego. While this is true, the yogi knows that behind these three is drishta (the seer or witness) and beyond that is the power of atman. While itself unmoving, atman is the source of the life energy that animates all the layers of our being.

Knowledge seems to come to us from outside, but on closer inspection a yogi sees that all knowledge comes from the self, as the capacity to know is the nature of atman. In the same manner, all peace and happiness come directly from atman and only indirectly by gratifying the mind and senses. The ancient sages discovered yoga by using different methods to unlock the secrets of atman. This is why yoga considers the investigation of one's own self (svadhyaya)

---

[2] One traditional definition of atman is "that which breathes." Atman is not one of the seven energetic centers or chakras that many yoga schools describe as underlying the function of body and mind. Nor is it one of the three subtle bodies (shariras) or five sheaths (koshas) that other schools say encase the soul. Atman is the immaterial aliveness around which these layers and levels of our being manifest. SK drew upon all these yogic models, each of which describes how the pure awareness and pristine energy of atman comes into causal, subtle, and ultimately gross or material form.

as the highest tool for growth. All the spiritual knowledge in the world can be gained by it.

Atman is the life element and it is through the power of atman that the techniques of yoga activate the body and mind. When these two aspects of our nature are made dynamic with the flow of life force, our higher consciousness is awakened. Yoga uses this conscious dynamism to create, protect, and multiply our health and well-being. That's why a yogi must continually ask, "What makes the brain and body go? What animates these inanimate objects?" It is atman that produces the movement, acting through prana the life force. What is significant is that atman, while itself motionless, is the source of all movement in the body and mind.

UNIQUE AND UNIVERSAL

Even a little exploratory practice will enable you to discern that atman has two primary expressions. Yoga calls the first of these *jivatman*, or the individuated self. This is the aspect of you embodied in a one-of-a-kind personality and an idiosyncratic mix of traits, talents, interests, and inclinations.[3] Yoga teaches that each of us comes into the world with a drive to express this distinctive, in-born nature (*svabhava*) in the gradual developmental process known to psychologists as self-actualization. Similar to the Western concept of soul, jivatman can be thought of as who you are as an individualized expression of life energy, the seed-self lying at the heart of your ability to grow into a vibrant embodiment of your innate capacities, and find fulfillment by walking your unique path in life.

Yoga calls the second aspect *Paramatman*, or Supreme Self, the aspect of you that is transpersonal and truly universal. (Paramatman is

---

[3] While expressing through the mind and body, the jivatman exists on a more fundamental level of reality than the character, personality, or ego and remains untouched by their deficits or conditioning. Some yoga schools refer negatively to jivatman as a bound soul because it easily gets hypnotized by the constant stream of sensations, emotions, and thoughts flowing through the mind, and as a result mistakenly identifies with the body. SK emphasized our ability to witness the activity of body and mind, which breaks this hypnotism and frees the jivatman to act consciously and creatively in the world.

one of many synonyms for Brahman.) Much like the western concept of spirit, Paramatman is unbounded and undifferentiated, a seamless unity that transcends the limits of individuality. Yoga teaches that each of us longs to recognize and remember this ultimate identity in a timeless moment of Self-realization. Paramatman can be thought of as what you are on the level of pure being, and its presence is the foundation of your ability to know complete and unfettered freedom.

> *Every living soul has two natures: penultimate and ultimate. The first takes the form of a body, mind, intellect, ego, and unique temperament. The second is identical with the power by which the whole universe is maintained. There is no separation in the conjunction of these two natures; there is only an appearance of duality. Cold makes water into ice, and heat makes it into steam, but water is water.*

Yoga places great emphasis on the fact that soul and spirit do not only meet in atman; they coincide. In other words, there is only one self, with two aspects that are distinct but not separate. It is this unity of imminent and transcendent that makes it possible for a yoga practitioner to access the cosmic power of Brahman and channel it constructively into a human life. It is this self-same unity of soul and spirit that makes it possible for a mortal and transient being to touch into the unborn and deathless, tasting a peace that surpasses mental understanding. How can the part possibly know the whole? Deep down it just does, a capacity intrinsic to being a part, and a reflection of the primal unity at the heart of existence.

While taking in these pointing-out instructions, don't get lost in ultimates or abstractions. Atman is simply what's alive in you: your essential self. You can learn to recognize atman as your true self because it is always awake and pure—a fountainhead of awareness existing upstream of the mind's conceptual right/wrong thinking. Like an upwelling spring, it is perpetually fresh and brimming with a joyous, creative energy. Untainted by all the mind's polarized thinking and repetitive patterning, it is unconditioned and whenever attended to leads to spontaneous and dynamic action. As SK taught, *Atman is the heart and soul of yoga. Whatever yogic* pathway you may follow, it will remain fruitless without a living link to atman.

OPENING THE DOOR TO SELF-DISCOVERY

While all of this may sound a bit esoteric, making contact with atman through the doorway of the sensorium is the best starting place to engage in practical yoga because it's this direct connection to your energetic source that renders the tools of yoga potent and able to deliver the full range of benefits their practice has to offer. Swami Kripalu saw the discovery of the still point at the center of the mind and senses as a threshold yoga experience that empowers a student to walk a sure path to self-actualization and Self-realization:

> *The Bhagavad Gita teaches that yoga practice can only begin after self-knowledge is gained. But who can rightly be called a person of self-knowledge? This is not a topic for argument; it is a matter of yogic experience. It may be said that a person who considers the motionless atman to be the true self has self-knowledge. Such a person is able to witness all the activity of the body and mind. What a wonderful experience! One who knows this inaction at the heart of all activity has found the path of yoga; there is no doubt about it. Only after crossing over to this stage will a yogi's inner journey not be cut short by various obstacles. While there are many yogic pathways, this experience is the secure entry point for each and all of them.*

After being introduced to the idea of atman, it's normal to feel that you understand the concept but are not quite sure of how to put it into practice. All you need is a little guidance about the process of self-discovery. The operative word here is *open*. Simply open your mind and heart to the presence of this innate but forgotten spiritual source. You might imagine yourself standing before a long-locked door. Establishing a receptive attitude is the key, as once the door is ajar fresh air and light will immediately stream in. Turning the knob, you're likely to find the door a little stuck. But that's okay because yoga provides the perfect tools to nudge it open.

When done with an intention to open the doorway of self-discovery, the coupling of postures, conscious breathing, and meditative introspection is more than exercise. It's a revitalizing practice that aligns every level of your being with your true self, enabling you to consciously receive the inflow of source energy that sustains the body and empowers all forms of action. As the door of self-discovery swings open, you'll grasp the essence of yoga, not just mentally but experientially, and are likely to find yourself eager to undertake its practice.

> *Knowing the science of yoga makes the spiritual path easy. There is only one divine power in the body, but it functions differently in different organs and nerve centers. When it functions in the eyes, visual images are seen. When it functions in the ears, sounds are heard. When it functions in the nose, fragrances and odors are smelled. When it functions in the tongue, different tastes are experienced. When it functions in the skin, tactile phenomena are felt. When it functions in the brain, the mental capacities of thinking, reasoning, and memory occur. By doing correct and systematic yoga practice, this power that flows from atman is stimulated. First the yogi gains freedom from disease, and then all his capacities blossom. This enables his individuality to be fully expressed, and such a person quickly meets with success. Not only that, he experiences bliss and manifests his spiritual potentials. In short it is through stimulating this divine power that a yogi becomes fully developed.*

BE A DISCERNING STUDENT

Contemporary yoga is based on a view that philosophers call monism.[4] All forms of monism distil existence down to a singular essence that is

---

[4] The term was coined in 1728 by German philosopher Christian Wolff based on the Greek word *monos* (μονάς) meaning single. Many ancient Greek philosophers taught that everything in nature emanates from "the Monad" or "the One," variously described as a transcendent being, essential principle, or primordial substance. Monism now refers to a wide range of philosophies that view everything as originating from a unified source that exists on a foundational level of reality distinct from its diverse expressions. · This circled dot diagram was used by the Pythagoreans to represent the Monad, which they saw as the dot of Absolute Being at the core of existence from which all relative realities emanate. The yogis developed a similar and more-nuanced model—see chapter 11.

seen to express in multiple ways through a universal set of natural laws. Materialistic Monism asserts that matter is the ultimate reality. This is the view of twentieth-century science, which sees consciousness as an epiphenomenon of matter and seeks to explain all mental processes through the laws of chemistry, biology, physiology, and neuroscience. Yoga is an example of Idealistic Monism. It asserts that consciousness or spirit is the primary reality and sees the material universe as an orderly expression of its primordial and all-pervading intelligence. Monism is often contrasted with dualism, the view that reality is composed of two fundamental forces existing in opposition to one another.

Many early yoga schools viewed the world as the interplay of spirit and matter in the same way that traditional religion sees the world as a battle of good and evil. Few of today's yogis subscribe to this dualistic perspective, believing instead that all pairs of opposites spring from a primordial unity, a particular monistic view called non-dualism. Non-dualism became an integral part of the yoga tradition after the sage Shankara established his school of Advaita Vedanta in the ninth century. While Swami Kripalu affirmed the existence of an absolute reality (Brahman) that was singular and transcendent, he also accepted the tenets of dualism, and considered both views integral to the practice of yoga.

> *After entering the highest samadhi, the ancient yogis declared a great principle. In truth there is only omnipresent Brahman, which is entirely without attributes or form. This idea can be simply understood. We all know that electricity can do many things. It can generate light and heat, or freeze water into ice, and power all sorts of movements. So the idea that the entire universe could be an expression of an unseen spiritual force makes sense.*
>
> *Once there was a great yogi named Shankara who traveled all over India debating pundits, scholars, and philosophers to establish this principle of "advaita" (literally "not-two") throughout the land. While expounding his teaching of Advaita Vedanta, he acquired thousands of disciples who sincerely accepted this correct view of non-duality through logic. Yet that mentality did not enable them to see the all-pervading Brahman, which cannot be seen with the physical eyes.*
>
> *As long as the mind is active and experience is being received*

through the medium of the senses, we will see the world of form with all its different qualities. The only way to know the non-dual wisdom is to practice "dvaita yoga," which means the yoga with duality in it. If we look inside ourselves and think clearly, it will become obvious that there are two primary forces from which our life unfolds. One is the awareness of the mind or chitta. The other is the energy of the body or prana, which activates the senses. These two forces flow into us from our spiritual source (atman), which is a seed sown in us by nature. If we cultivate this seed by practicing the dualistic yoga of awareness and energy (the yoga of chitta and prana), it will become a tree with a strong trunk, many branches, and countless leaves and flowers. But a tree doesn't appear all of a sudden. When first planted, it begins as a small sprout and must grow in stages. Yet in every seed there is the potential for the great tree of a realized life.

It is through this two-fold yoga that we learn to control the senses and can speedily move through all the stages of self-development that make up the spiritual path. When this yoga finally takes us beyond the dualistic mind, we can enter into samadhi and see for ourselves that the ultimate reality is one without qualities and form. It is easy to say the drop of the jivatman merges into the ocean of Brahman, but you must understand what this really means. Yes, duality no longer exists. But non-duality no longer exists either. Even existence does not exist. At this point, there is no one left to tell someone else what to believe!

The teachings of Advaita Vedanta are considered the highest expression of the yogic scriptures because they are focused exclusively on ultimate truth. But dualism and non-dualism are both correct in their respective stage of practice, and it's important that you not get lost in the wrong stage. This is why I say a little at the start about Brahman to give your practice a right direction but after that emphasize the dualistic yoga of body and mind. That is the practice that enables you to fulfill your aims in life while progressing toward Brahman. Return to the teachings of Advaita Vedanta only when you have risen beyond thinking in your meditation.

APPLYING THIS CHAPTER IN PRACTICE

Even when practiced systematically and in accord with its guiding principles, yoga is at best a subjective science. It's not possible to objectively verify SK's claim that yoga brings you in touch with the power that created, sustains, and keeps the universe evolving. However, you can easily locate the power source he was pointing out by following the instructions that open this chapter. With a little practice, you can learn to regularly access this deeper dimension of your being, the pristine presence that underlies all sensory and mental experience, and draw on the energy you find there to cultivate the spiritual seed of the true self. You can do what SK did—earnestly conduct the experiment of yoga—and then assess its results.

Scholars of comparative religion say that every spiritual path presents a diagnosis and cure for the human condition. I believe that yoga would diagnose the root cause of all our difficulties as a break in connection with our spiritual source. Yoga's remedy is to restore this connection to full vitality, using it to nurture the health of body and mind, and end the self-alienation that leads to so many of our problems. Everything else, including the realization of the highest non-dual truth, is best seen as a by-product of that revitalized connection.

The important and early role of self-discovery in yoga practice is illustrated by this traditional Indian story, which likens the spiritual path to a pious pilgrimage upon which the importance of this lesson is learned right at its outset.

TEACHING STORY: DON'T DISCOUNT YOUR SELF

Ten young men came together from neighboring villages to make a pilgrimage. On the first day they planned to follow dirt roads until they came to a wide river. Once across it, they would spend a week traversing a network of paths up the Himalayan foothills. Arriving at the base of a tall mountain, they would ascend to its summit where a sacred temple stood. After offering prayers, they would return home to share any insights or blessings resulting from their efforts.

The group set out early the next morning. Hoping to reach

the river before nightfall, they maintained a brisk pace and only stopped briefly for lunch. Evening was approaching when they discovered the bridge across the river had been washed out by a recent flood. Eying the calm waters, the group decided there was enough light to wade across, which would enable them to spend the night on the far bank.

Forming a line, they entered the river and soon found themselves chest deep and fighting a swift current. At times it seemed certain that all ten of them would be swept away. Emerging on the other side, they fell on the ground exhausted. Darkness came quickly, and it was all they could do to eat their food uncooked and fall asleep.

Early the next morning, the group leader woke with a start. Seeing his sleeping comrades, he counted them one-by-one to make sure everyone had made it across the river. Finding only nine bodies huddled around him, he uttered a loud gasp. This woke up another of the pilgrims, and the leader told him, "Look at our group—I count only nine—one of us must have been lost to the river." Starting with the group leader, the second pilgrim counted the others one-by-one. He also found only nine. Soon everyone was awake and lamenting the lost group member. A plan was hatched to break into two groups and go down both sides of the river. If he could not be found alive, they would at least recover the body.

Just then an old swami was passing by. Seeing the men and alert to their agitation, he asked, "What is the matter?" The group leader explained, "Yesterday ten of us set out on pilgrimage. Now we are only nine. One of us must have been swept away last night while crossing the river." The swami saw immediately that there were ten young men standing before him. He asked the group leader to show him exactly how he had counted. After hearing his answer, the swami declared, "Rest assured, the tenth pilgrim is alive!" The group became silent and the leader said, "Did you see him on your way here?"

"No," the swami answered, "You are the tenth pilgrim. You forgot to count yourself!" Having learned this lesson, the men returned to their pilgrimage and were able to successfully complete it.[5]

While expressed in a humorous fashion, the moral of this story is deftly stated. Don't discount the power of your own self! I was fortunate to learn a portion of this lesson early through a defining moment in little league baseball. At twelve years old, I was the catcher for the Hollidaysburg Braves and we'd made it into the playoffs. In the first round, we faced a team from a nearby agricultural area called The Cove. Most of their players were farm kids with little baseball experience, but they had ridden into the post season on the shoulders of their ace pitcher, who was a man among boys. His name was Glenn Hostetter. As he warmed up on the mound, his biceps looked bigger than my thighs. All the way from our dugout, we could make out the shadow of his developing mustache. In the background was the banter of our parents, who were questioning whether this young buck was truly thirteen and eligible to play.

We batted first, and it only took a few pitches for our entire team to fall into shock. This guy threw the ball at a speed that rendered it invisible. Our leadoff hitter was his first strikeout victim. I was next in the lineup and proud of my batting average. Four pitches later, I was back on the dugout bench without taking a single swing. Along with blazing speed, Glenn had the control required to pound the strike zone. In the first three innings, he mowed down our entire lineup as fastball after fastball whizzed into their catcher's mitt. Other than a walk or two, we couldn't get a guy on base. But they hadn't scored a run either, so the game remained a zero-zero tie.

It was late in the game when I stepped into the batter's box for the third time. Whether he threw me balls or strikes, I was determined to go down swinging. I decided to begin my hitting action early, just as Glenn was completing his windup. The first pitch whizzed by same as before, but trying to hit it gave me some sense of the ball's whereabouts. That was important as up to then I was just trying to get lucky. Now I believed there was some chance I could make contact with the ball. I could tell the second pitch was right down the center. My timing was off,

---

[5] This story was known in the ashram. Although there is no record of SK telling it publicly, I'm confident it was part of his large repertoire of teaching stories.

but it felt like I'd come close. Trembling, I said four life-changing words to myself. "I can do this."

The third pitch came and I swung at the blur. A crack of the bat sent a low line drive up the middle. When the center fielder bobbled the ball, I was on base with a double. Then a miracle occurred. As soon as the barrier of impossibility had been crossed, one after another of my teammates were able to get hits. Enjoying a late rally, we easily won the game. This experience changed me. Facing a seemingly impossible situation, I had refused to stand there with the bat in my hands. I didn't give up. And by making an effort, I'd succeeded.

This is the first time I remember when the willingness to believe in myself generated an inflection point in my life, but it was far from the last. I've found countless instances where simply viewing something as possible and making a start turns out to be the defining factor in success. It was not all that different when I came to the ashram and grasped the real purpose of yoga. How could a kid from the boondocks of central Pennsylvania possibly discover the invisible power of atman? While this endeavor would take considerably longer than a little league baseball season, I kept believing in myself and eventually made contact.

The path of yoga is often presented as an arduous uphill trudge in which every level of your being must be purified before any chance of standing on the mountain top of Self-realization exists. As a novice practitioner, I adopted that view. Looking back, this was a major league mistake, and one that you as a reader can avoid. It's not true—or even logical—that a person needs to struggle the better part of a lifetime for Self-realization when the core of their being (atman) is innately whole, spiritually-connected, and awake in this moment. Yet our conceptual viewpoints have the power to not only frame but determine our life experience.

If yoga is viewed as an iffy and painstaking proposition, the idea of an arduous path to enlightenment will become a self-fulfilling prophecy. But if yoga is viewed as a natural process of bringing forth the essential self that is already fully-formed within you, and eager to express, your practice will swiftly carry you forward. Seen in this light, the process of ripening into Self-realization may take time to gain momentum, but the moment in which the fruit will drop of its own accord becomes inevitable.

None of this is meant to imply that victory can be declared after a superficial self-discovery, or that a genuine depth of Self-realization is easily gained. While both of those statements are untrue, the most advantageous view of the yogic path is one in which self-discovery easily occurs at its outset. This enables you to begin touching into moments of self-recognition, and start living and practicing yoga as that connected Self sooner rather than later. Remember those four magic words: I can do this!

A yogi in quest of Brahman takes pleasure in exploring the core of their own being (atman). Truly, an aspirant who does not perform this continued practice of self-investigation (atman vichara) strays from the path. As declared in the revealed teachings: Let the yogi introvert the senses to meditate on the light of the Absolute Brahman shining in his own soul as atman, for this is the path of yoga and the highest refuge.

CHAPTER 5

PURUSHARTHA: THE FOUR AIMS OF LIFE

The sole purpose of yoga is to help you achieve the four aims of life: dharma (a way of living that truly works), artha (material prosperity), kama (pleasure and enjoyment), and moksha (liberation from all forms of suffering and the freedom to express yourself in dynamic action).

Yoga is not meant to be a speculative pursuit. On the contrary, it's a sure bet that if you engage its disciplines while focusing on your inner source you will get more energy. I sensed this at the outset of my practice. Studying Swami Kripalu's teachings, I gained an understanding of it. Forty years later, it remains a daily truth that I rediscover each morning on my mat and cushion. As this foundational promise of yoga becomes a reality for you, it will lead you to ask an important question: "What am I supposed to do with this energy?"

After your interest in yoga is aroused, you will explore some practice and experience an exuberance of energy all over your body. Your face will light up with pleasure. Your mind will become sharp, and your intelligence will approach brilliance. Feeling that life is worth living, you will be motivated to shed old habits, succeed in new self-efforts, and attain your maximum development. This is the secret of yoga.

He answered this question by coupling yoga practice with an Indian philosophical doctrine called the four aims of life. According to the yogic sages, humans are born with four motivating drives that emanate directly from the soul (atman). Each drive exerts a steady pull of desire that gives rise to what the sages considered a noble pursuit because if acted upon properly it will enhance your life and also benefit others. Yoga as taught by SK is a pragmatic science that empowers you to find fulfillment in an active quest to meet each and all of these four aims.

> *In yoga there are four goals in life, which together are called purushartha. Purusha means "soul" or "individual being" and artha means "goal." Each of us has many goals, but yoga consolidates them into these four categories, and all of our desires can be listed under one of these basic pursuits. The purusharthas reflect the universal and perpetual needs of human beings. Without reflecting upon them, it is not possible to begin true yoga practice, which is a path of spiritual upliftment through which individuals attain happiness, families and communities prosper, and everyone contributes to the welfare of the world.*

Dharma, artha, kama, and moksha: understand these terms and the interrelatedness of the powerful drives they reflect, and you will be able to channel the energy generated by your yoga practice into a purposeful life.[1]

DHARMA

Consciously or not, we are all on the lookout for a trustworthy way to avoid problems and achieve success. We instinctively monitor the environment, alert to threats and opportunities, but also gauging the results of our actions to learn from the subtle interplay of cause and effect. Our ears perk up at new ideas and more nuanced ways of thinking that augment

---

[1] The Indian doctrine of purushartha appeared in a set of texts called the Dharma Sutras (aphorisms on dharma) written between 300 BCE and 100 CE. It was fully developed in the multitude of teachings stories told in the Indian cultural epics of the Ramayana and Mahabharata. The first three aims can be conceptualized as emanating from jivatman or the embodied soul. They motivate us to meet our biological needs, pursue our purpose in life, fulfill our personal dreams and desires, and apply our talents to maximize our contribution to society. The fourth aim arises from paramatman or spirit, which calls us to discover that aspect of our being that is transpersonal and desireless. Serious yoga practitioners often believe that they should have no wants or needs, a presumption this teaching says is not only mistaken but impossible.

our understanding of how the world works. We draw upon that understanding to act in a purposeful manner that meets our needs and keeps us on good terms with the social environment that surrounds us. All of this reflects what SK called the drive for dharma, which is considered the first and foremost of the four aims for an important reason. Deep in the human psyche, more essential than the desire for sex, power, or possessions, is a longing for a true state of security and fulfillment that leaves us always on the search for life orienting knowledge (dharma-vidya).[2]

Dharma is a keystone concept in yoga and a word with no English equivalent. It's impossible to provide a single definition, as the term has a long history and evolved over many centuries to reflect a nuanced understanding of what it means to engage in a right way of living, one that can be relied upon to produce positive results because it is aligned with the flow of natural forces and the way things actually are, or truth. Recognizing this drive for dharma explains why yoga considers everyone at heart a truth seeker, as each of us is constantly striving to refine the fit of our worldview to reality.

Yoga's teachings on dharma originate from an organizing principle simple enough to often go unstated. Everything in existence emanates from a singular source of intelligence and power. If you attune to that source and endeavor to live in harmony with it, you will naturally act in ways that meet your immediate needs, unfold your potential, and positively contribute to society. But if you disregard and live in dissonance with that source, you will run into endless difficulty. The symptoms of what yoga calls adharma (not-dharma) are clear: aimlessness, apathy, addictive patterning, and the malaise of self-alienation. The indicators of dharmic alignment are equally clear: life makes sense and living it day-to-day feels meaningful and worthwhile. When all aspects of a yogi's dharma slot into place, the energy of the cosmos pours through them, illuminating their minds and empowering their actions to a startling degree.

[2] On the path that SK taught, dharma-vidya (understanding the principles of right and successful living) leads to yoga-vidya (understanding how the techniques of yoga are meant to be applied) which ultimately leads to Brahman-vidya (enlightening and liberating knowledge). Psychology as a whole emphasizes the physiological drives such as hunger, thirst, sex, and comfort. Humanistic psychology also recognizes the drive to grow in self-awareness and attain self-actualization, which is tantamount to yoga's drive for dharma. The drive for spiritual awakening and liberation or salvation has been the exclusive province of religion until recently when the emerging field of transpersonal psychology began investigating it.

Dharma can mean law, religion, morality, ethics, civic duty, cosmic order, or life purpose. Understood properly, it's a mindset that integrates all of its many definitions into a "discipline of right action" that brings a practitioner a balance of life's four aims. The Ramayana puts it this way: "In this world, all material gain and happiness are to be found in the pursuit of dharma. From dharma issues both profit and pleasure. One attains everything by dharma, which is the true strength in this world." The Mahabharata expresses the same view a little differently: "It is from dharma that all prosperity and enjoyment flow. Neither for the sake of pleasure, nor out of fear, nor due to greed, should one abandon the principles of dharma."

In truth we all have the power to succeed in life, but only if we connect ourselves to atman. First the practice of yoga remedies bodily diseases and removes ordinary miseries. Controlling the senses becomes easier, which makes our mind more composed and joyful. As vices start to fade and virtues develop, we feel drawn to live dharmically and our spiritual power steadily increases. Radiating energy, people are drawn to us and it becomes possible to act skillfully to accomplish the three personal goals of life. Eventually we are motivated to seek the fourth and final goal of liberation. Truly this path of dharma is the shortcut to success.

When Swami Kripalu spoke of dharma as the search for happiness, I believe that he was pointing his Western students back to the ancient Greek philosophers like Aristotle. Aristotle taught that all human beings strive for *eudemonia*, a state of well-being and flourishing. He called eudemonia "the whole aim and end of human existence," a solitary good "desirable in itself" with all the lesser amenities of life sought to further this primary goal. It was classical ideas like this that seeded the cultural rebirth of the Renaissance and flowered in the European Enlightenment. The early Enlightenment scientist and theologian, Blaise Pascal, said it this way: "Man wishes to be happy, and only wishes to be happy, and cannot wish not to be so."

Drawing on a host of Enlightenment thinkers, America's founders helped usher in the modern era by declaring everyone's right to life, liberty, and the pursuit of happiness. Two and a half centuries later, we live in a culture obsessed with the idea of happiness. Most of us pursue it earnestly through hard work and the career advancement needed to acquire all the necessities and nice touches that we believe will make our lives worth living. As consumers we fuel a global economy with a worldwide standard of living that has never been higher. Unfortunately, so are the rates of anxiety, depression, substance use, and suicide. Why is the sense of comfort, ease, and feeling good in the moment that we associate with the word happiness so hard to hold onto?

Like the philosophers of old, SK knew the Goddess of Happiness cannot be courted directly. Anyone taking this tack only finds her running in the other direction. Yet happiness can be sought in a way that doesn't dead end in materialism or spiral into existential despair, but instead leads to our ongoing growth and development. The roots of this approach to well-being are cross cultural and deep. What Aristotle called the way of virtue, SK called the path of dharma. If we dedicate ourselves to this discipline of right action, sages East and West declare that the Goddess of Happiness will come seeking us.

In the depths of our heart, we are all looking for happiness and to find it we must be free to pursue our chosen aims in life. We know this from the history of slavery. Many slaves had stern masters who treated them violently. They were worked continuously and not given enough food or sleep. But other slaves were given these things and still they wanted to run away. Where an animal might have been satisfied, a human being is an altogether different entity. To be able to express their humanity, an enslaved person will gladly take a mountain of troubles upon their head and even face death. In modern times, we have this freedom, but right living has become defined as that which results in wealth and fame. This definition is incorrect, and for anyone following it lasting happiness is not possible. In the yoga of ancient India, right living is defined as that which results in the elevation of the mind, character, and collective culture. This is the path of dharma that brings forth the higher qualities present in every human being. Following it, one can reliably attain health, prosperity, knowledge, true fulfilment, and a spiritual bliss that otherwise remains out of reach.

This discipline of weaving together personal and societal good is dharma's defining feature, and SK's teachings explain how our individual needs can be met in a way that makes the world a better place. The next few chapters delve into dharma's most important definitions with an eye to how its principles can be applied in life. All you need to know at this juncture is that dharma is the first aim of life, a right way of living meant to bring everything you need to flourish.

Students who start the practice of yoga with proper guidance will awaken life energy and have many positive experiences. If they take up the mantle of dharma, they will benefit from these experiences. Set on the path of progress, their life energy will remain active and they will continue to practice with great enthusiasm. Students who do not give importance to dharma will fall prey to adharma and its many vices. Overridden by problems and difficulties, they will lose faith and their inspiration will come to an end. It can be said that a person's progress along the path of yoga is directly proportional to their commitment to right living.

ARTHA: SECURITY AND PROSPERITY

The second aim of life is *artha*, a word that means wealth but refers more broadly to the drive to establish a livelihood that meets our survival needs, grants a measure of material security, and bestows a feeling of prosperity. Artha is best seen as incorporating all the resources needed to fulfill our duties and purposes in life. This includes basic needs like food, clothing, shelter, owning the tools of one's trade, transportation, and the financial wherewithal to cover routine expenses. It also includes a stable supply of less tangible resources like physical vitality, mental focus, and a sense of freedom from scarcity and lack.

Yoga does not equate artha with material goods alone. Many other things are also valuable and rightly considered forms of wealth and prosperity. From a yogic perspective, we should treat our bodily health, mental well-being, our capacity to give and receive love, our practical know-how, and our higher knowledge as precious assets.

What it takes to satisfy the drive for artha will vary from person to person in accord with their circumstances. A family man or woman needs to sustain a stable home environment. Later in life, they are likely to face the financial challenge of simultaneously sending kids to college while saving for retirement. A business leader at the helm of a growing company may move in social circles where a degree of affluence is not only expected but essential to success. A solitary artist may choose to live frugally to maximize their free time for creative pursuits. To be wealthy in yogic terms is to have an abundance of whatever you need to fulfill your aims in life. Aristotle expressed this eloquently: "He is happy who lives in accordance with complete virtue and is sufficiently equipped with external goods, not for some chance period but throughout a complete life."

Yoga was developed by forest dwelling monks and nuns whose religious vocation was best served by an austere simplicity. As a result, it is often identified with a minimalist mindset. This mistaken view reflects a renunciate bias that curtails yoga's scope of usefulness. SK recognized that everyone has material needs and respected the role that meeting them plays in a well-rounded life. This is evident in the prayer with which he routinely ended his public lectures: *May everyone here be happy. May everyone be healthy. May everyone be prosperous. May no one be the least little bit unhappy at all.* He also taught:

If yoga was solely a means of realizing God, then it would only be of value to seekers of liberation. Yet everywhere in the world householders are living with spouses and children who rightly desire wealth, status, prosperity, and power. Dharma is the only means of honorably gaining these attributes of happiness, and it can truly be called the yoga of everyone. Even if its practice is followed only a little by individuals, their progress is assured. Through its proper performance by society, humanity could truly manifest heaven on earth, not just externally but internally in the heart of each person.

As a monk, SK owned little beyond his clothing, pocket watch, fountain pen, and personal library of sacred texts. But he needed regular meals, and a peaceful place to do his practices, along with the financial backing of influential people to accomplish social projects central to his life purpose and aimed at improving the lot of everyday people. Free of any judgment that being affluent was unspiritual, he was comfortable moving among the higher classes and enlisting their support. Teaming up, they were able to provide a wealth of food, education, vocational training, and medical care to those less fortunate.

Research has proven the terrible toll that poverty, and the relentless stress that comes from lacking needed resources, take on people's health and well-being. Above the poverty line, studies show that income is positively correlated with happiness, with a nest egg of savings providing an important buffer against misfortune. While people are happier with money than without it, the research also confirms the old cliché that money alone can't buy happiness. Significant hikes in per capita income across the globe have only resulted in modest increases to empirical measures of people's overall life satisfaction. Once a person's material necessities are covered, the data suggests that their focus shifts to satisfying higher needs.

KAMA: ENJOYMENT

We all long for something more than safety and security. The third aim of life is *kama*, which is often translated as pleasure but better defined as enjoyment. The good life is not only secure and stable; it's comfortable and joyous. Kama begins with sensory pleasures like appealing food and sex, but quickly extends beyond the body to embrace our psychological need for intimacy, friendship, fun, and adventurous new experiences. Along with the sense of belonging that comes from supportive family and friend relationships, it includes the higher pleasures of intellectual learning, skill acquisition, creative expression, and all the myriad forms of accomplishment. Instead of self-denying, the yoga taught by SK affirms our drive for physical comfort, emotional warmth, and enjoyment as a noble aim of life.

The concept of kama conveyed by the Indian sages mirrors the pleasure principle espoused by Sigmund Freud that originated with the ancient Greeks. We are instinctually wired to seek pleasure and avoid pain. This motivating drive is nature's way of prompting us to meet our biological needs. Its force must be understood and respected as a vital component of our evolutionary guidance system. Only then will healthy efforts to discipline the body and mind bear fruit. It might be surprising to hear that SK believed *the best way to resolve a cherished and life-enhancing desire is to satisfy it*. But he considered the corollary to this principle equally important: *Chasing after distracting, trivial, or harmful desires wastes energy and is often a source of pain. They are best set aside and allowed to wither.*

If desire is not cast in the role of a spiritual enemy, a yogic life can be rich with the pleasures of wholesome food, loving relationships, comfortable and beautiful surroundings, creating and appreciating art, and all sorts of intellectual avocations. On top of the interludes of enjoyment this provides, a person deriving genuine joy and satisfaction from daily life will have the staying power required to persist through difficulties and accomplish their larger and long-term goals.

> *Dharma is that which raises the individual, the family, the nation, and the whole world to a higher level. By its practice, the beastly and self-serving in us gets replaced by a humanity that goes on developing step-by-step. It is dharma that enables us to fully participate in society and find meaning in earning the money required to support our families. It is dharma that allows us to gain enjoyment by fulfilling our cherished desires while also maintaining a harmonious relationship with the whole universe. Truly, it is only through a commitment to right living that we can be victorious over obstacles and grow into a real human being.*

It's important to underscore that SK was not teaching that happiness can be gained simply by accumulating wealth or indulging our senses. What the Greeks called hedonism, yoga calls *bhoga*, or pleasure seeking. Anyone operating with this mindset quickly discovers that desire is insatiable. When one craving is satisfied, another quickly arises to take its place, often accompanied by a general feeling of discontent. In its worst expression, the cycle of desire and gratification can become greatly amplified in the physiological and psychological phenomenon of addiction.

An astonishing amount of energy can be generated by a steam engine. Similarly, an extraordinary energy is generated in the body of a yogi by practicing self-restraint and right living. Bhoga is the inferior path of sense-based pleasure seeking that leads to the descent and loss of this energy. Yoga is the superior path of spiritual elevation that leads to the retention, ascent, and sublimation of this energy into good behavior, happiness, accomplishment, and the climax of samadhi. Bhoga is thus the antonym of yoga, while the synonym of yoga is brahmacharya (defined below).

SK knew that it's easy to squander the energy generated by a regular yoga practice in frivolous pursuits that sidetrack us from our deeper purposes. To avoid this pitfall, he stressed the need to combine yoga with a lifestyle of moderation that enables vital energy to build to high levels where it can uplevel health, empower creative action, and catalyze psychological growth. The importance of moderation in a yogic way of life is reflected in the name the Indian sages bestowed upon it: *brahmacharya*, which means "the vehicle that will carry you to the ultimate good" (Brahman).

In my practice, I've learned that food, sex, physical activity, productive work, and sleep are not just biological needs. They are outlets I use to manage my energy. As more energy flows into my system, it takes self-awareness and a healthy dose of self-discipline to channel it wisely. At various times, all these areas of my life have gotten out of balance as I've passed through the embodied learning process of yoga. Over time, I've come to recognize the truth of what psychologist Mihaly Csikszentmihalyi says on page three of his groundbreaking book, *Flow*: "The way to happiness lies not in mindless hedonism but in mindful challenge.... The best moments of our lives are not the passive, receptive, and relaxing times. The best moments usually occur when a person's body and mind are stretched to its limits in a voluntary effort to accomplish something difficult and worthwhile."

The energy of a yogi practicing under the protection of dharma is always increasing. This rouses the inner spirit and generates new hope, new enthusiasm, and inspires new actions that evolve the mind and body. The progressive raising of one's energy is how suffering can be overcome and happiness gained completely from within.

Psychologists have shown that we are born pleasure seekers, with infants preferring sweet tastes, comforting textures, and harmonious sounds. Research also confirms that pleasurable experiences including eating, sex, and recreational activities that release tension and reduce stress are strong components of adult happiness. The only problem with pleasure is that it is fleeting. Satiation comes quickly, and exceeding its limits brings dullness, boredom, and pain.

Everyone can practice yoga and travel on its path of spiritual well-being. The first objective of a yogi living in society will be health, wealth, family, and worldly success. A yogi fulfills these aims, not necessarily by having more and more, but by deeply understanding their role and duties in life, and accepting the need to develop themselves to accomplish their goals. When after many years such a yogi realizes the heights of human fulfillment, they also see the limitations of advancing their material welfare and having fun. At that point they will naturally take recourse in the outer path of service and the interior path of meditation as the means of gaining true peace and joy.

MOKSHA: LIBERATION

By legitimizing the role that passion, pleasure, and material prosperity play in life, the four aims invite us to channel the power of our instinctual drives and psychological desires into an integrated system of personal growth and spiritual awakening. Yoga practitioners operating within the riverbanks of dharma are free to raise their energy and engage wholeheartedly in a quest for fulfillment. Along the way, they are sure to cultivate virtue and grow in wisdom. SK praised ambitious people who traverse this first leg of the yogic journey and achieve what he called *success in life*:

In India, a person who fulfills their life's true mission is called "siddhartha." This is a beautiful name that has a secret meaning.

> "Siddha" means "accomplished" and such a person has made the effort to accomplish the first three aims of life or "arthas" and by so doing has become fit to pursue the highest aim of moksha. It is not by chance that the Buddha's given name was Siddhartha Gautama, as he was destined to grow beyond these aims to seek moksha and become one of the great light bearers of our world.

Over time, life teaches all of us that a lasting happiness cannot be found in transient things. While praising dharma, SK made sure his students understood that the culmination of yoga entails more than health, wealth, self-expression, and all the goods he grouped under the rubric of *human fulfillment*. It requires knowing firsthand that we are more than our mortal body and limited mind, which can only come from directly experiencing the unlimited and imperishable ground of our being (atman/Brahman). This is the essence of the fourth aim of life, which the yoga tradition calls *moksha*—liberation.

In the deepest regions of our psyche, we all yearn to see beyond the boundaries of the human condition and find release from the confines of our day-to-day existence. All great art and literature speak to this longing. In much the same way that we instinctively seek bodily pleasure, we have an inborn and irrepressible hunger for rapturous and transcendent experiences—insights, epiphanies, and revelations of all kinds. Yoga teaches that our thirst for these mystical experiences is rooted in a single imperative—the need to progress along a path of development that positions us to discover who and what we truly are. And much in the same way that bodily hunger and thirst informs us of the existence of food and water, yoga teaches that there is a specific type of experiential knowledge able to satisfy our heart's deepest yearning.

While in some ways a fourth and final goal, moksha is qualitatively different from making efforts to satisfy the first three aims of life because these peak experiences tend to only occur when the strategizing activity of the thinking mind that underlies all our goal-directed striving ceases. In that breach and opening, a special type of gnosis or knowledge can enter us that both yoga and Buddhism describe as being beyond-the-mind-and-senses (*atindriya*), which is said to grant an intuitive understanding of the true nature of the all phenomena (*prajna*).

> *There are four efforts sanctioned by the Indian scriptures with the fourth (moksha) being the pursuit of ultimate liberation and freedom. On the path of yoga, the aspirant following dharma and the aspirant seeking moksha are both standing on the same bank of the river of existence. And yet there is a difference between the two. The aspirant seeking liberation has awakened the desire to go across the river.*

For most yogis, the practical expression of moksha lies in those seemingly serendipitous moments when our sense of separateness falls away and the essence of us shines through in a clear-seeing consciousness unburdened of fear and untainted by mental filtering. Even a passing taste of this beyond-mind state can spark a spiritual awakening that heralds a course of positive change. The kind of repeated glimpses that occur in a regular meditation practice, or even a single strong experience, can bring about the overall change in being signified by the term Self-realization, which is a precursor and milepost on the way to the completely-realized state of moksha.

> *Whenever direct knowledge of the Absolute is obtained, the mind becomes disengaged. This cancelling of the mind is the doorway into moksha. As long as the mental faculty remains active, the externally-directed senses will continue to carry on their various activities. Only when this action ceases can the yogi enter samadhi and realize the deepest truth. This cancelling of the mind is the one and only means of attaining liberation. Those who do not consider mind-cancelling to be the key to liberation do not know yoga.*

Current research is shedding light on the neurobiology associated with these unitive experiences. In depth meditation, it appears the brain's neural networks that enable us to locate ourselves in space and time are switched off, while the networks that keep us present and paying attention remain active. Temporarily freed from our ingrained sense of being a separate, skin-bound individual, we experience ourselves as connected to everything and everyone around us. Scientists are confirming what yogis and mystics have long known. These moments of communion and union inject our lives with a profound sense of meaning that markedly increases our happiness and resilience.

> *Liberation practice is a special kind of worship. After the yogi attains control over the senses, the activity of the mind is slowly extinguished. Mind gradually becomes no-mind and the yogi becomes free of the bondage of the body. As sugar melts and completely disappears in milk, the mind disappears into nature. This is moksha, which bestows everlasting peace.*

In traditional yoga, senior students were encouraged to make an all-out effort to stabilize this experience of unity consciousness through ardent meditation. Their solitary aim in life became moksha, a positive state of transcendental knowing said to bring about *dukkhanta*, the cessation of all forms of misery and sorrow. SK guided all his students—except a handful of renunciate swamis—to progress toward moksha gradually, letting the path of dharma ripen them spiritually until an intense and wholehearted longing for liberation spontaneously arose and naturally shifted their life focus.

I've learned that it's best not to conceptualize moksha as a final goal only attained at the end of the spiritual path. Any insight or inner shift along the way that clarifies our perspective on life and liberates us from some portion of our suffering can rightly be celebrated as an expression of moksha. This positive view is a much-better traveling companion than spiritual striving, which allows for precious little joy in what is meant to be a lifetime journey. For me at least, the daily sense that I am growing and evolving in the direction of an ultimate good is a big factor in my overall happiness quotient.

BE A DISCERNING STUDENT

The sage's four aims of life are remarkably similar to the needs hierarchy propounded by Abraham Maslow in 1943. Over the next quarter century, Maslow helped found the academic field of humanistic psychology and his needs hierarchy became one of the most influential models in the behavioral sciences.

Maslow describes people as motivated to meet a progressive set of survival, security, belonging, self-esteem, status, and self-actualization needs. Where yoga's four aims lump many important areas of human endeavor into the single category of *kama*, or enjoyment, Maslow's broader grouping is more current and helpful. Yet Maslow's final goal of self-actualization, which is accomplished by developing the capacities of our egocentric self, falls short of expressing our full spiritual potential.[3] Arguably, this potential is better conveyed by the yogic concept of Self-realization, and taken together these two models provide a solid intellectual basis for the approach to yoga taught by SK.

APPLYING THIS CHAPTER IN PRACTICE

I embarked on the path of yoga as a rebellious youth coming of age in the afterglow of the 1960s. Like many in my generation, I was seeking an alternative to materialistic values and consumerism. At first, I was disappointed to find SK advising me to pursue security, pleasure, and *success in life*, which seemed little more than a spiritual makeover of the normal American mindset. I didn't know then what I can now say for sure. This was the conceptual framework I'd needed to understand how yoga's principles and practices fit together to form a coherent approach to life. Walking the path it charted would transform my consciousness while bringing me the best of everything life has to offer. But before that could become a reality, I had to get clear on my life purpose, another aspect of dharma and the topic of the next chapter.

---

[3] Near the end of his life, Maslow attempted to amend his famous theory to include a top tier of development called "self-transcendence," which he said can be gained by "tapping into the resources of that aspect of our being that lies beyond the individualized sense of self." Approaching his death from a heart condition and experiencing this higher level himself, Maslow grew adamant that a person should not get hung up at self-actualization. In the same way that it was limiting to not rise above the lower developmental levels focused on safety and security, he felt that self-actualization can become its own limiting prison. In the aftermath of Maslow's death in 1970, the significance of this final stage in his life, and the crowning stroke to his needs hierarchy it produced, was overlooked and tragically never added to his influential model. Had this change been made, Maslow's model and the four aims of life doctrine would be entirely consonant. For more on this story, see the book *The Finders* by Dr. Jeffery A. Martin.

Wherever yoga is practiced systematically, health improves and character development occurs. Prosperity, pleasure, divine revelation, and salvation naturally follow.

CHAPTER 6
SVADHARMA: YOUR LIFE PURPOSE

Dharma is a word foreign to you but its meaning can be said simply. Dharma is a way of living authentically in this world that imparts great purposefulness and true happiness to anyone applying its principles.

Dharma is packed with meaning, which explains why this single word has so many differing definitions. Broadly speaking, it is a right way of living meant to carry you successfully through life. But dharma has other important connotations including the one spotlighted in this chapter: your mission or purpose in life. The key to unpacking the full meaning of this multivalent term is to know that taken together all of dharma's definitions chart out a developmental progression. Answer the call of dharma by putting its principles into action, and you'll find that each one becomes especially apt and applicable at a particular juncture of your yogic journey.

What Swami Kripalu called *the path of dharma* has a definite starting place as efforts to proceed from anywhere else inevitably go awry. This inception point is *svadharma*, which means "one's own dharma."[1] The sages explained the concept of svadharma in lofty metaphysics, describing how everything in existence arises from an underlying field of pure intelligence. They envisioned each of us as an individual soul (jivatma) conceived as a noble idea in the cosmic mind of God (mahat) and imbued

---

[1] Literally, self-dharma. This old idea lives on in popular religious thought and its echo can be heard in the message of the contemporary lay theologian, Michael P. Kassner, "You are a unique person called into being because, without you, something would be missing in God's masterpiece called Creation."

with a novel point of view, a practical purpose to fulfill in the world, and some enduring quality that contributes to the wholeness of humanity. In the eyes of the sages, this soul-self is who you truly are. Their overarching guidance is to resist the suppressive force of conformity and bring this authentic self forward to accomplish your purpose in life (svadharma). Only by doing so can you grow into a mature expression of the person you were born to be. They saw this as the only way for individuals to fulfill their destiny and society to truly flourish.

As an Indian scholar and spiritual teacher, Swami Kripalu was intimate with the term dharma and used it often and in varying contexts. The result was that any single use of the word could mean a right way of living, a person's guiding purpose in life, yoga's framework of moral and ethical principles, or any other of its many connotations. Even while studying his lectures closely, I often found myself confused as to which facet of dharma he was referring.[2] I would never have understood the central role that a person's life purpose plays on the path of yoga without the help of Aristotle, whose well-reasoned argument on how to attain happiness was easier for me to grasp.

ARISTOTLE ON PURPOSE

Aristotle begins his argument with the assertion that "nature creates nothing without a purpose." Just as the purpose of the eye is to enable us to see, the purpose of the hand to allow us to grasp, and the purpose of the foot to grant us mobility, the whole of a human being must have a reason-for-being over and above that of its parts. Aristotle then asks his readers to ponder: "What is this purpose?" He argues that a real answer has to involve more than sustaining life, as even plants do that. Nor can

---

[2] SK did not group his teachings on life purpose under the subheading of svadharma. Nor did he use the subsidiary term sadharana dharma, which means "the ethical principles applicable to all," and is the topic of the next chapter. Only after recognizing these subcategories, and seeing how he focused upon them at different places in his teachings, was I able to sort things out. I am not implying that SK used the word dharma loosely or in a thoughtless manner. The same problem is encountered studying Taoism and its primary text the Tao Te Ching. Much like dharma, the word *tao* can mean the way, as in the path followed by a Taoist sage, a way of living that is in harmony with nature, an ethical way of conducting one's self in relationship to society, and the way the universe works. While any single use of tao might highlight a particular facet of its overall meaning, all its definitions are to be held in mind at once, not as alternatives but as an integrated whole.

it be limited to accurately perceiving the external world and following the prompts of instinct to satiate the senses, as animals do that quite well. It has to be something more distinctly human than either survival or pleasure seeking. Aristotle urges us to contemplate this question deeply because hidden in its answer is an important secret, as nature bestows happiness on anything that truly fulfills its purpose.

This is where Aristotle's thinking gets nuanced and interesting. He accepts the practical reality that humans are communal beings who need to produce a diversity of goods and discharge a multiplicity of functions to live in an orderly society. In meeting these collective needs, he recognizes that individuals are not alike. They have differing dispositions and talents, which adapt them to performing different occupations, with society best served when its labors are divided up and performed by individuals skilled in a particular area of expertise. Therefore, he reasons that we should exercise care and choose a line of work well-suited to us.

Aristotle acknowledges that a happiness peculiar to humans comes from performing our chosen occupation well and working hard to make a meaningful contribution to the collective welfare. Writing thousands of years ago, his words still ring with relevance. A cobbler should strive to make comfortable shoes, and a carpenter to build soundly. A sculptor should aspire to express beauty, a harpist to sound the notes of harmony, and a geometrician to ascertain not merely the approximate angle that may suffice for the carpenter, but the precise angle befitting a mathematician. Whatever craft, art, science, or manner of business you perform, do it purposefully and with excellence. And if possible, over the course of your life, make some contribution that advances your field of expertise, as human society only progresses through the efforts of innovative individuals who find ways to increase our common knowledge.

But Aristotle's argument does not end there because human beings share a deeper and more vital purpose. The true function of a man or woman is not only to perform their activities "well and rightly," but to steer the course of their entire life with intentionality, exercising all their bodily, mental, and spiritual faculties wisely and in conformity with the ennobling ideal of virtue. This is the essence of what it meant to be a philosopher or "lover of wisdom" and someone dedicated to expressing their knowledge in wise action. Aristotle advises us to "Live a life of total virtue, as to be truly happy takes a complete lifetime. For the return of one swallow, or a single fine day, does not make spring. Similarly, a day or brief period of happiness does not make a person supremely blessed and happy."

> *I have grown in knowledge by studying books on philosophy. Such study must include contemplation, which is the churning of intellectual knowledge by philosophical reasoning. But a yogi cannot accept the truth of even a great philosophical argument by study alone. True knowledge only comes when you complete this process by conducting personal experiments in which you put the argument to the test by applying its component principles in your life.*

Aristotle concludes his argument with an authoritative statement. Only to the extent that you fulfill these purposes in life will you know happiness. He then advises anyone interested in following the way of virtue on how to find their calling. "Where your gifts, talents, and abilities intersect with the needs of the world, there you will discover your purpose. These two, your talents and the needs of others, are the great wake-up call to your true vocation in life. To ignore them is in some sense to lose your soul."

I was mesmerized by Aristotle's argument, in part because SK's disparate teachings on dharma contained all the same elements, and I could now see how they fit together. Like Aristotle, SK starts out by making the point that human beings are something more than animals:

> *Dharma exists in a human being in the same way that heat exists in fire. Without heat, fire doesn't exist. Without dharma, a human being doesn't exist. Animals and humans share a common need for safety, food, rest, and sexuality. Where the actions of animals are prompted by instinct, humans have the capacity to think, reason, exercise restraint, and act consciously. This is a special attribute of humans. Without a dedication to dharma, we are animals without horns and tails. We simply eat, sleep, urinate, defecate, and reproduce like any other animal. You may not agree with this statement, or be uncomfortable with it, but this is the view of yoga. It is*

dharma (the principles of right and ethical living) that enables us to recognize the power of our animal nature, see how it can either enslave or liberate us, and choose to act in ways that enable our personality and humanity to develop beyond it.

He continues with the idea that people are not alike. Each of us has a distinctive self-nature (svabhava) that gives rise to a one-of-a-kind personality and unique way of being. A trustworthy life path must respect the role played by individual differences, as a one-size-fits-all spirituality will only lead us astray.

Everyone has their own nature and temperament, which gives rise to our different inclinations and interests. From ancient times, yoga has recognized that human beings are of three primary types. Some are intellectuals, others emotional, and still others display an action-orientation. But many of us are not predominantly one or the other. Our nature is a mixture of these types. We also may have some distinctive quality that gives rise to our specialness and is important to recognize. Given all these individual differences, how are we to find our way forward in life?

It is in all of our natures to move in the direction where we find attraction. If those attractions are acknowledged and cultivated, they grow stronger and liking begins to take place. Liking gradually increases and becomes self-knowing. This knowing is unique in character. It takes each individual in a specialized direction. Just as animals learn how to run, fish gain the ability to swim, and birds discover how to fly, we can follow our liking to find a way to move along the path of life that is natural to us.

In daily life, we are free to choose a line of work to pursue. In our meditation room, we can experiment with different techniques. Sage Patanjali says that no matter what work or practice we may choose, it is yoga if done with concentration. This explains why it's necessary to have a natural attraction for whatever it is that we choose to do. The mind can only concentrate on tasks that it likes and is interested in doing. Any successful person, when asked how they attained to their goal, answers: "Through concentration." As lovers of yoga, we should keep this in mind and strive for mental steadiness in all our activities.

Then SK makes a point about our flaws, foibles, and personal struggles that Aristotle does not mention but I've found important enough to highlight here.

There are two more things an aspirant must know about his or her nature. In the same way an automobile has both a forward and a reverse gear, our nature includes some areas of weakness. These are the birthplaces of our harmful habit patterns, and we must patiently work to overcome them. Only after we have triumphed in this struggle can we look upon these areas and see them as beloved kinsmen. Truly, these are not enemies or even impediments, but the source of our greatest attainments. Also, we must not expect to be skillful in our dharmic actions as soon as we start performing them. Before we gain the expertise required to arrive at our goals, we will have to continue our efforts despite failing many times. This inevitably requires great patience and perseverance.

What is my nature and how must I conduct myself in order to become successful in my life? Dwell on the above principles and think this question through carefully. Be specific and accept only those thoughts that you like and feel drawn to establish deeply in your mind. Then make a sincere effort to apply them in your daily life, while also practicing the techniques you enjoy in your meditation room. Acting in this way, your nature will express itself more and more powerfully. It is this yoga, which recognizes the differences in each aspirant's nature, that produces the best results.

Swami Kripalu didn't speculate much about the source of our inborn self-nature. At times, he referred to the accepted psychological principles of his day, or quoted authoritative yogic texts. If alive today, he'd likely mention nature and nurture along with the emerging science of genetics. Instead of trying to explain this mystery, his focus was pragmatic in encouraging each of us to come into a greater awareness of this idiosyncratic nature that influences so much of our behavior.

We all have experienced taking an immediate like or dislike to certain activities, domains of thought, or individuals, without any obvious reason. Even though we do not know where these likes and dislikes come from, we find that we cannot easily rid ourselves of them. Psychology explains this mystery by saying these likes or dislikes come from our past experiences and the unconscious mind. The Bhagavad Gita speaks to reincarnation and karma. It is the duty of everyone to become conscious of their own nature and use it to achieve happiness, peace, and joy. Accepting this self-nature is the only way to acquire knowledge from the rich storehouse of the soul, and the sanity it bestows will eventually lead us to work for the good of others.

He goes on to describe how each person's nature interacts with their circumstances in life to give rise to the guiding purpose signified by svadharma. This purpose is not something we create tabula rasa as if we start out as a blank slate. It's hardwired into us from birth and accompanied by a corresponding set of interests and aptitudes that when cultivated become critical life skills. In the same way the blueprint for an oak tree is instilled in every acorn, the seed of an authentic and purpose-driven life lies hidden in each of us. Once this seed has sprouted, it will continually generate new growth. Where drumming up motivation is a constant problem for a person conforming to meet externally-imposed goals, an individual intent on discovering and doing their svadharma awakens a soul-force that enables them to ride a wave of creative passion through life.

In today's yoga world, the idea of svadharma is sometimes reduced to the search for a socially-responsible job that can legitimately be considered "right livelihood."[3] What we do to earn our daily bread is certainly an important part of the equation, but equating svadharma with career robs the teaching of its real power. Svadharma is an orientation meant to inform the whole of our life including personal relationships, family

---

[3] Right Livelihood is one step on the Buddha's eightfold path, which he defined in the sixth century BCE as avoiding "evil trades" such as soothsaying, ones involving trickery, usury, or trading in weapons, living beings, meat, intoxicants, or poison. In positive terms, it is earning your living by "right and honorable means."

matters, civic duties, and recreational pursuits. Aristotle and SK both used the term vocation in its classic sense as a strong inclination or calling to pursue a particular course of action and line of work in life. When this is understood, the Bhagavad Gita makes perfect sense when it says: "It is better to engage one's own dharma and perform it imperfectly, than accept another's vocation and perform it perfectly. Misfortune may be avoided by undertaking the duties prescribed by one's own nature." (chapter 18, verse 47)

> *Dharma arose in India, but its teachings do not exist to change your dress, external behavior, or even your thinking. Dharma's only aim is to bring forth those divine qualities already present in you but lying dormant in the soul. This is the foundation of any living religion, which exists purely on a spiritual level, and the seeking out of these innate qualities is the true search because only through them can you attain to an authentic, unshakeable, and virtuous way of life on this earth. Real dharma requires tremendous freedom, as it does not seek to make you a follower of any faith. Instead, it points to the individual nature and favors self-knowledge as the means of growth. Other approaches are less enchanting and will only help avoid external temptations. The way of dharma enables you to hold fast to your self-chosen vocation and not lose heart despite difficulties galore.*

Swami Kripalu didn't recommend an intellectual approach to students wanting to identify their true calling in life, perhaps because he felt that was likely to result in paralysis by analysis. Instead, he suggested a simple way to feel your way forward by noticing what activities light you up with positive energy, and then giving yourself permission to move in that direction.[4] He also told the story of his early life when depression dogged his attempts to follow in the footsteps of his deceased father, who had worked as a municipal bureaucrat. That was before he

---

[4] For an inspiring exploration of this topic, see *The Great Work of Your Life: A Guide for the Journey to Your True Calling* by Stephen Cope. For those needing help in identifying their svadharma, *The Four Desires: Creating a Life of Purpose, Happiness, Prosperity and Freedom* by Rod Stryker offers a systematic approach.

spent a year-and-a-quarter in his guru's ashram being schooled in yoga's approach to right living.

When his time of ashram tutelage abruptly ended, SK was forced to return to his hometown and set his adult life and svadharma into motion. He was a novice aspirant on the path of yoga, this much was obvious to him. But he had no interest in becoming a swami. The thought of living off alms was repulsive to him. From childhood he had a passion for literature, and was a gifted writer with musical talent, but doubted whether he could develop any of these skills sufficiently to make his way in the world. After a period of soul searching, he launched an unlikely career as a poet and dramatist, and the rest of his life unfolded from there. He walked an authentic path in which he was a playwright, music teacher, Sanskrit instructor, sought-after public speaker, humanitarian, and eventually a renowned yogi. All of these roles and stations reflected his guiding purpose in life, which evolved over time and shone ever more brightly.

SK ON FINDING YOUR SVADHARMA

You can come to know your seed purpose by noticing whenever your body and mind naturally become cheerful. At first just try to discover whatever caused this good cheer. Then make an effort to stabilize its presence by doing this dharma daily, and by so doing remaining joyous and happy. When a person recognizes their most important purpose in life, their life expression must go through a powerful transformation. A seed planted in the ground ruptures before it begins to grow. Many obstacles arise on this first branch of yoga. Do not be afraid or disappointed by them. Through the medium of yogic practice, you can be victorious in any field. Simply persevere in this purpose until you attain your aims and goals. Those who excel on this path know fulfillment and are likely to become popular, prominent, and prosperous.

We all walk a path from birth to death, but there is no way to describe an individual's movement through life in general terms. That's because the life of each individual is colored by its special aim and purpose. Unless that special aim is given expression, our journey will remain vague, a drab sketch of what our life could be. If we seize upon that aim, all colors become available to us in its painting. It's only in viewing many such paintings, each by a different artist and distinct from all the others, that a true portrait of what human life is can be seen.

Everywhere Lord Krishna is recognized as one who has completely mastered yoga. He was born to rekindle the light of dharma in society at a time when the world had grown dark. That was the purpose of his incarnation, and his life story symbolically reflects it. From early childhood, he possessed an enchanting nature. His endearing smile and mischievous actions enticed not only his mother but all the women in the village to pour their love into him. As a young man, he was very out-going and dressed differently than others. His garment was made of yellow cloth, a most unusual color in those days. He wore his headdress a little crooked and adorned it with peacock feathers. Today we might say that he was a fashion-plate.

As an adult, all of Lord Krishna's duties were carried out in a distinctive manner that demonstrated his energetic effervescence and skillfulness. This is why one of his names is Chel Cha Bilo, which means "a person who is expressive in all his dealings." He was not trying to impress anyone. He was simply expressing his self-nature. As a result, its enchanting power kept growing and through it he was able to accomplish his important mission in life. You too can do this.

BE A DISCERNING STUDENT

It is almost an article of faith in spiritual circles that anyone intent on awakening beyond the egocentric self must forego personal ambition. There is a logic to this. Highly awake individuals throughout history—like Jesus, Buddha, Ramana Maharshi, Ananda Mayi Ma, Mohandus Ghandi, Martin Luther King, Jr., Nelson Mandela, Mother Teresa, Vimala Thakar, and in our time Mata Amritanandamayi—display surprisingly little concern for comfort, wealth, status, or the trappings of worldly power. They are accurately characterized as having transcended the egocentric self, whose grasping for outer validation only reinforces its sense of being needy, separate, and apart.

Given this fact, the way to become more like these great souls seems clear: act to weaken the individualized identity. Acting on ideas like this, aspiring yogis often develop a mistrust of their motivating drives, channel their energies in circular or push/pull patterns of behavior, maintain ambiguous boundaries in their relationships, and express their spirituality by striving to "kill the ego." In the process, they often short-circuit their self-development and sabotage their own success.

While it's true that highly awake individuals display what could be called "selfless traits," this line of reasoning may not accurately reflect how they got there. If you study their lives, it becomes evident that individuals of this stature have tremendously strong personalities. Instead of being alike, they are decidedly different, and in their actions display a trait that psychologists would ironically call ego strength. SK exemplifies this pattern, as it was his ambitious early life that ripened him for a powerful mid-life awakening. Perhaps that's why he openly encouraged students to question the approach of discounting the individualized identity.

The Upanishads say the weak attain neither worldly success nor God. A yogi must contemplate this statement. If a weak-willed person cannot even attain the material goods needed to survive, how can they reach the summit of spirituality? We all begin the practice of yoga with a polluted mind. There is ego, selfishness, and many things that make us ask, "What can I really accomplish here?" Even under such trying situations, if we practice the techniques of yoga they will purify us stage by stage. Our power starts increasing and we can secure the material conditions we need. We soon see that propagating the ego is not going to bring us real success, which requires the clarity born of mental peace, so our practice grows subtler and begins to refine the mind. Negative samskaras (impressions and patterns) are purged and positive potentials are actualized. As these positive traits take over the mind, we cease efforts to build up the ego, and it begins to melt away. In yoga there are many meanings and stages of the word "self." One is "ego" but the highest is "atman." The best way to dissolve the ego is to develop our humanity, which frees our authentic self to come forward and attain its aims in life. Yet this higher science of mind and self does

> *not stop there. It goes on increasing and eventually brings forth our divine potentials to ready us for realization and emancipation.*

In practicing the yoga SK taught, one of your primary tasks is to inquire deeply into your purpose and calling in life. Only then can you align your inner drives around that purpose, using the tools of yoga to energize your self-system. Instead of weakening your sense of self, this approach enlivens your personality with life energy. It empowers you to walk a path of self-expression in which the satisfaction of your basic needs is a step on the way to realizing your highest aspirations. That's what the word authentic signifies in the context of yoga: a self-aware person who knows what is theirs to do and is comfortable being who they naturally are while doing it.

APPLYING THIS CHAPTER IN PRACTICE

Make no mistake! People who take the road less travelled confront many challenges. Conforming to the expectations of others is easier, but a thoughtful person has to question whether it presents a viable long-term path to happiness. Living as anything less than one's true self seems bound to lead to apathy, depression, the bitterness of resentment, and ultimately regret. While inspiring new students to explore and endeavor to achieve their life purpose, Swami Kripalu never cast the path of dharma as a stroll in the park.

> *Consciously or unconsciously, the quest for happiness is the daily pursuit of everyone. Yoga philosophy says dharma is the true path with the power to remove all forms of unhappiness, after which only happiness remains. But yoga philosophy also acknowledges that an army of hardships surrounds each and every person. Most of these hardships are dormant, but whenever given a chance they become active and hurl their unhappiness upon us. This is why the Bhagavad Gita teaches that anyone born into this life has to be a warrior.*
>
> *Unless you are willing to battle this army of hardships, your survival, success, and liberation are impossible. Under these circumstances,*

it's easy to run this way, then that way, anxiously searching for a way to escape the conflict. Dharma is standing firm in your purpose and duty, remembering that none of these hardships has the power to interfere with your destiny. The pain of struggle is real, but the sweetness of the great happiness experienced at the end of all these lesser unhappinesses is indescribable.

I graduated from college feeling like a lost soul. My passion was yoga, but back in the early 1980s I could not see any viable way to make that front and center in my life. I completed my law school applications in despair, bowing to parental pressure because I didn't know what else to do. While studying for the bar exam, I made a small but significant decision. Instead of joining a law firm, I took a position as a staff attorney in a legal aid office representing senior citizens and indigent clients, a job more aligned with my values. Over the next five years, I did my yoga early each morning and during the day acquired the skills that prepared me to eventually become Kripalu Center's lawyer, a position I held for a quarter century.

Serving through Kripalu Center's fiery transformation from a guru-led ashram to a nonprofit educational organization was not an easy assignment. After that startup phase was behind me, handling the legal work of a bustling guest center required long hours, and I was often asked to wear multiple hats. Everyone involved in shepherding the Center into a stable nonprofit business had to live with a great deal of risk and uncertainty, as it often felt like one threat or another would topple our guest-house of cards, and it would be lights out for the organization's mission and the end of all our livelihoods.

Looking back, the form of my svadharma was never static. Danna and I were physically present at Kripalu whenever I held high-level administrative roles. At other times, I was able to work remotely from our home in Virginia with monthly trips back and forth to the Berkshires. On numerous occasions, it seemed my usefulness to the organization had run its course. Readying myself to look for other work, some next iteration of my role was always proffered.

From where I sit today, I am amazed that it all worked out. Kripalu Center became the largest yoga-based retreat center in North America, affording Danna and me the opportunity to serve in a setting that supported our practice. Living simply, we were able to save enough to fund a modest retirement. Svadharma was not a philosophical concept to us. It was tangible, something that we worked at every morning on our mats and cushions, and continued all day long at our desks, which kept both of us engaged and on the whole happy. All these years later, new leaders have come forth and Kripalu's doors remain open, something that means a lot to us.

Highlighting our story may make it seem that svadharma is a teaching aimed at young people, or those lucky enough to work at a yoga center, but I don't think that is accurate. As adults we all need to stay attuned to our life purpose, feeling out those things that are uniquely "ours to do." While career is pivotal, so is family life, with friendships and avocations providing outlets for self-expression. Danna was a public librarian and archivist for decades, writing each morning after meditation, before blossoming as a poet and publishing her first book. Be always on the lookout for whatever will keep your creative juices flowing, and find some way to do it.

Both Aristotle and Swami Kripalu believed that an enduring happiness was always hard-earned over the course of a lifetime. Here's a simple but symbolic story SK told to illustrate his teachings on svadharma that inspires us to walk our self-chosen path despite the peanut gallery taunts and painful hurts we're bound to encounter. It is easy to see how our highest nature is reflected in the compassionate saint. It's less apparent that our lower nature is also depicted in the aggressive scorpion.

TEACHING STORY: THE SAINT AND THE SCORPION

Once a saint with an unusually kind and gentle nature was bathing in the river. Submerging himself, he came to the surface and noticed a large scorpion a little upstream that was being pulled away from the shore by the river's current. Feeling this poor insect would die, and knowing very well that it had a powerful stinger, he started wading towards the scorpion. Cupping his hands, he made an effort to get some water along with the scorpion and toss both onto the riverbank. Despite his effort, the scorpion was able to sting him. The saint's hand recoiled and the scorpion landed mid-way in the water. So the saint stepped close and took the scorpion in his palms a second time intent on throwing him to safety. But again the scorpion stung and the saint's toss failed to reach dry land. Several people had gathered on the shore and shouted, "Swami, why are you doing this? The scorpion is not going to give up his violent nature." The saint replied, "When this ordinary animal will not let go of his nature, even when facing death, why should I abandon my nature, which is to help him?" A third time the saint caught the scorpion in his hands and threw it toward the shore. The scorpion also showed its strength, stinging the saint even harder than before. His whole hand burning, the saint felt ecstatic seeing the scorpion fall onto solid ground and scuttle off to safety. This saint was a mahatma—a great soul—but all of us must suffer stings if we want to stay true to our spiritual nature and svadharma. Such pain only lasts for a short time, where the joy that comes from expressing our soul self in life is enduring.

CHAPTER 7

SADHARANA DHARMA: THE ETHICAL PRINCIPLES APPLICABLE TO ALL

The great masters of yoga have proclaimed a universal dharma that condenses within itself the ethical principles of all the world's religions. The success achieved by influential men and women across various fields is invariably founded upon their practice of one or more of these principles. This dharma is meant for everyone regardless of ethnicity, nationality, social class, or stage in life. Those ignoring this spiritual science are stunting their own development.

While I wanted to be a good person, the topic of ethics never held much appeal. Growing up in the 1960s, I pushed back on any externally-imposed rules that blocked me from doing what I wanted. I brought this libertine attitude with me to yoga and remember my first encounter with its shortlist of ethical precepts. There were five behavioral restraints. Based on my Catholic upbringing, I interpreted them as thou shalt not's: non-violence, non-lying, non-stealing, non-indulgence (or moderation), and non-attachment. These were followed by a matching set of prescribed observances or in my mind thou shalts: purity, contentment, study, self-discipline, and surrender to the Divine. It's not that the list was lacking. I just wasn't looking for a code of conduct to steer my life by. I wanted to be more spiritually-connected, self-directed, and spontaneous in my actions. So I skipped right over the restraints and observances to get to the real stuff of postures, breath control, and meditation.

I'd been practicing a few years when I realized that Swami Kripalu looked at these precepts in an entirely different light. Instead of limiting constraints, he saw ethical conduct as the means to get what he wanted, legitimately and in a way that catalyzed his self-development. The 180-degree clash in our perspectives piqued my interest. It led me to carefully scrutinize SK's teachings on dharma. Eventually I was able to distil his yogic prescription on how to succeed in life down to a single sentence. Energetically pursue your purpose (svadharma) and aims in life (purushartha), while honoring the ethical principles applicable to all (sadharana dharma). In other words, set your sights on what you really want and go for it, acting consciously and in a way that is morally and ethically sound. It was only after this light bulb turned on in my mind that I became eager to put these precepts to the test.

> *A person who starts doing yoga becomes happy but soon feels that practice alone is not enough. That's why yoga gives us a set of guidelines to follow that make all facets of our life an art. It includes behavioral restraints that remove obstacles to our growth, and ordained actions that enable us to realize our highest potentials. If we try to live within these guidelines, we stay happy. If we disrespect them, we are visited by unhappiness once again. Sisters and brothers, if you've decided to walk the path of yoga, accept these guidelines right from the start. That way your mind will become peaceful and you will grow spiritually in your meditation room. While laboring amidst the chaos and difficulties of your workplace, your mind will remain composed, enabling you to pass the tests of daily life and advance in society. This is the way to satisfy your desires and progress spiritually too. Honoring the restraints and observances may seem arduous, but fear is unwarranted, as you are only required to practice them to the best of your ability.*

Swami Kripalu credited the yogic sages with an important discovery. In deep meditation, they intuited that the natural laws governing the cosmos include a universal set of ethical principles. The sages taught that anyone wanting to raise energy and access higher consciousness must align with these principles as the evolutionary forces of nature will only flow powerfully through a well-intentioned person seeking to better themselves and serve the greater good. That's why yoga includes techniques designed to develop us morally and ethically. While wrongdoing may in some way leapfrog us temporarily forward, it inevitably creates inner dissonance, generates outer conflict, and boomerangs back in surprising ways to torpedo our success.

> *It is inaccurate to think of dharma as a lovely idea thought up by an intellectual. Dharma is a gift of the yogis, who gained insight into how life actually works. The natural laws discovered by science cannot be destroyed. Even if the knowledge of gravity is everywhere forgotten, it continues to exist and operate. Yoga is such a science, only most people have not become aware of dharma and its secret principles. Where a good person practicing ethics will meet with ordinary success, a yogi practicing dharma will become a great being and meet with extraordinary success. This statement reflects the power of yogic science, but its accuracy can only be verified by conducting the experiment. The water of a river flows between two banks, which ensure that it is always progressing toward its goal of the ocean. A yogi's life is also a river, flowing toward its aims between the protective banks of the restraints and observances.*

Informed by these teachings, my experience of the restraints (*yamas*) and observances (*niyamas*) began to change. Instead of rules to follow, I began to sense how these principles were alive in me as the roots of my conscience. They palpably reflected something stirring inside that wanted to come forth more fully, a kinesthetic kind of integrity totally different from being a goody-two-shoes. But before this could happen, I had to confront what felt like a stone wall of cynicism blocking those roots from sprouting to the surface. My mind was convinced that any effort to adhere to all these ideals was sure to render me straitlaced and ineffectual. I didn't want to be a timid, milquetoast yogi. I wanted to be powerful in my life. I honestly could not tell whether my reticence was well-founded or a defensive mental ploy to keep me from embarking upon the path of right action. All I knew was SK believed that it was not only possible but pragmatic to embody these principles.

Danna made me a calligraphy list of the restraints and observances, which I framed and hung in our yoga room. Every morning before exiting, I would pick one to reflect upon during the day. The effect of this exercise was totally unexpected. Holding an ideal like non-lying in mind, I was forced to watch myself diluting and dissembling from the truth at every opportunity. This reality check on my righteousness quotient was daunting. For a time, the list loomed large in my mind. Even looking in its general direction brought mental anguish. The best I could do was try to keep myself from violating its ten principles in egregious ways.

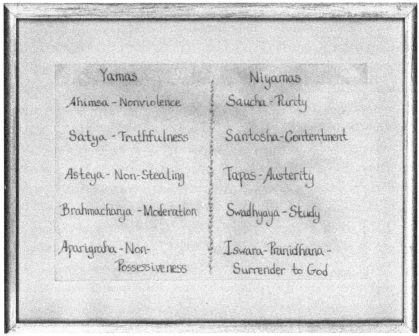

Danna's shortlist of the five restraints and five observances prescribed by the Yoga Sutra. SK drew from the full library of yogic texts to arrive at a comprehensive list of twenty-three virtues—see Chapter 17.

As month after month went by, I was amazed by how little this consciousness-raising practice did to reform my conduct. Despite my good intentions, I kept right on doing and saying all sorts of things that were unwise and less than true. Watching my life play out against the backdrop of yama and niyama, I had to admit that the lion's share of trouble I encountered was self-generated.

Morality remains superficial unless it is connected with the roots of our being. That's why yogis do more than read scriptures and ponder philosophy. They practice techniques to forge this connection, which enables them to express the principles of dharma in their thought, speech, and action. Thinkers who believe themselves great moralists and continue to act in an egotistical manner are called hypocrites. They lack the mix of humility and courage required to attain self-knowledge. Only when our good thoughts are reflected in our words and deeds can it be said that we have unblocked the pathway to our success.

My practice remained rudimentary until it dawned on me that SK was not using the term dharma to describe a static system of morality and ethics, but rather a fluid developmental progression. This insight sparked a breakthrough, as it enabled me to see that a scrupulous right/wrong mentality was not the end point of the frustrating path along which I was crawling. Gradually I was able to discern in his teachings the outline of a step-by-step training that heretofore had not been apparent. Morality was an initial step, important in itself, but also a stepping stone toward exactly the kind of self-directedness I was seeking. This upped my motivation considerably.

Full-strength religion requires a direct connection to soul and cannot be practiced by everyone right away. Morality is its inception, but that is only religion's outer husk. Halfway between morality and true religion is the practice of ethics, which is based on the purest of principles (the restraints and observances). Always remember and never forget that a virtuous character is the only pathway to a living religion and through it alone can true spirituality be attained.

The first of these definitions of dharma is law. Choosing to follow the rightful rules of society requires impulse control and exercising it stimulates moral development.[1] Modern life is complex and complying with all of its do's and don'ts can leave a person feeling rule-bound. While the notion of being an outlaw might sound romantic, studies show the inability to curb instinctual urges is a profound barrier to happiness and success. SK minced no words in saying that each of us has a duty to overcome our brutishness. He saw morality as the bond underlying

---

[1] A yogi also follows nature's "laws of health" to create harmony in the body and mind, a topic addressed in chapter 14.

an orderly and just society, as well as a foundation every yogi must put in place and never abandon as they move on to explore more of their human potential. By strengthening their moral backbone, a yogi gains self-respect and earns the trust of others, acquiring a social currency only granted to those with the self-discipline needed to abide by accepted norms.

Today I will talk about dharma. Dharma is often described as morality or religion, but the correct Sanskrit word is "satachar." Sat means truth and achar means to practice. So dharma is defined as practices that align us with the truth of how life works

While pursuing their aims and interests, a yogi must constantly ask: "Will this action or thought take me closer or farther away from truth?" This is because yogis know that dharmic acts build energy and raise consciousness, and adharmic (contrary to dharma) acts dissipate energy and lower consciousness. It can be said that yoga is acting in accord with the moral and ethical principles of dharma to energize and elevate our consciousness.

All of us are subject to strong sensual desires and times when our fearing mind threatens to possess us. A yogi is one who struggles to purify the mind so it can resist our lowest tendencies. One who cannot forego wicked actions and make sacrifices for the happiness of his or her fellow beings is not yet ready to set out on the path of saints and spiritual masters. For one intent on moral conduct, this path effects a spiritual renaissance that replaces artifice with straightforwardness, restlessness with peace, enmity with love, poverty with prosperity, and self-centeredness with a genuine desire to be of service.

Dharma is life, and life is dharma. The two are not separate. If you want your family to be truly happy, you will have to practice dharma at home. If you want your business to be truly successful, you will have to carry dharma with you to the office. If you believe dharma lives in this book, you will remain in trouble. But if you apply dharma in whatever setting you find yourself, you will meet with success everywhere, because its principles reflect how life actually works.

Life is perpetual motion—it doesn't stand still and neither do we. True and lasting happiness comes when we move in the direction of progress. Pain and suffering come when we move in the direction of downfall. If humanity were to take up the practice of dharma, it could destroy all obstacles to progress and together we could manifest our hidden divinity. May we all become dharmic beings.

But at this point in my self-development, I was ready for dharma's next definition, ethics, and its application in a practice that SK called *character building*. Where morality relies upon restraint to check wrong action, ethics uses the power of positive actions to strengthen the good traits that undergird our personality. His approach to building character appealed to me. Instead of fighting with your faults and problems, channel your energy and attention into salutary conduct, allowing harmful habits to wither away. It was already evident to me that I was at heart a person who wanted to do the right thing. Sizing up the yogic virtues, I grew convinced that adopting them would serve me in many ways.

I have learned the science of character building from the scriptures, the biographies of great persons, the company of saints and masters, and my own experience. Its principles are the treasure of my life, which I freely dispense to others wanting to mend their lives.

The primary principle is that bad character traits can be eradicated by strengthening good character traits. By applying this single principle, you can formulate the best possible personality. It has a corollary that is equally important. Do not wrestle with a fault that you want to remove. Wrestling only increases the disturbance of the mind, which enables the excited fault to lift you up and slam you to the ground. Unable to pull yourself up to fight again, you will eventually give up the fight forever. The best way to remove a fault is to practice its opposite virtue, which decreases mental restlessness and increases self-regard.

Experience shows that anyone who personifies an enormous power of purposeful determination and excels in their chosen field is by necessity wedded to self-observation and virtues such as healthy eating, regular exercise, and yoga's restraints and observances. Master these virtues and you will also be successful.

Character building brings more than high-mindedness. A truly virtuous person wields a type of power and influence that arises from their commitment to values that transcend their own self-interest. They've become what SK called a *person of principle* who can act decisively because they have a guiding purpose, a working moral compass, and a set of ethical compass points with which to navigate. Embodying yoga's ethical precepts, they are like a boat with a keel in the water that trues them up and keeps them moving in the right direction. The practice of character building is presented in chapter 17.

Yoga's step-by-step training does not end with ethics. The last developmental definition of dharma is "being in tune with the universe," a condition sought through the practice of karma yoga. Where the twin disciplines of moral restraint and character building are used to uplevel our degree of self-control, karma yoga is designed to free a yogi from the limits of the dualistic mind and ego, making it possible to act intuitively as an instrument of spirit. Yoga teacher, Richard Miller, captures the sense of what this feels like in a pithy aphorism. For an adept karma yogi, "Each moment is paired with its perfect response." Where an ethical person stays true to principle, the actions of a karma yogi spring directly from their spiritual source. These spontaneous actions are imbued with the intelligence of the whole. As a result, they are prescient and carry the wisdom of paradox. Acting in a natural way that integrates all of life's polarities, a karma yogi flows easily through life.

> *Advanced yogis cease to feel that they are the doer of their actions. This is why Lord Krishna at the end of the Bhagavad Gita tells Arjuna to give up any concern for right action or wrong action and let his actions be entirely directed by prana (the life force flowing from soul). But this teaching of total freedom is the highest expression of yoga. Before it applies to us, we must examine ourselves honestly. Have I really given up wrong actions? Have I accepted the need to patiently do right actions for a long time to foster mental purity and steadiness? Have I grown to the point where I am truly able to decide what I want to do, and what I don't want to do, and act accordingly without any attachment to the results? Have I done enough actions without attachment to exhaust the potent samskaras (subconscious impressions) that motivate unconscious*

behaviors and generate conflict in my life? Only when we have risen to the heroic level of Arjuna in our yoga can we understand and apply the concluding teachings of the Bhagavad Gita. Until then, we should carry out our everyday duties skillfully, ethically, and with great love.

Swami Kripalu admired Mahatma Gandhi for walking the path of character building and karma yoga to its full expression. As his autobiography makes clear, Gandhi conducted himself in accord with yoga's restraints and observances even while spearheading the movement for Indian independence. Guided by the Bhagavad Gita's teachings on karma yoga, he was able to remain mentally at peace in the face of extreme political pressures and threats to his life. In the end, it was Gandhi's ability to act spontaneously and intuitively that confounded the British and helped his country win its freedom from colonial control.

As a student and practitioner, I found it necessary to tease apart SK's teachings on morality, ethics, and karma yoga. But he didn't draw rigid distinctions between them. Instead of separate domains, he saw them as slices of a single developmental spectrum in which morality matures into ethics and flowers in karma yoga. For him, everything comes to a yogi committed to treading the path of dharma:

Every yogi knows that when we try to sit in stillness any wrong acts we have done arise and create a disturbance in our hearts and minds. Regardless of how talented we are in the art of meditation this will be the result. In order to quell restlessness and know tranquility, these acts—to the best of our ability—should not be performed.

The importance of ethics can be seen by the status it holds in every nation and all fields of human endeavor. Even in the domain of modern warfare, where it would seem that its practice would be impossible, ethical rules are set and respected. It is only the person who feels they are practicing the restraints and observances to the limit of their capacities who can cross the boundary from ethics to karma yoga.

Yoga tells us that we will be happy to the extent that we live in harmony with reality—this is the essence of dharma. And we will experience unhappiness as we grow further away from reality—this is the essence of adharma. When we grasp this fact there is no need for anyone to command us to observe dharma and forego adharma because we all want to remove suffering from our life. The energy of a yogi practicing dharma is always increasing. This rouses the inner spirit and generates new hope, new enthusiasm, and actions that further evolve the mind and body.

Do not give up dharma to meet minor or petty needs, as relinquishing its principles produces feelings of guilt and makes the mind unsteady, which interferes with reaching one's major life goals. Greatness awaits anyone able to exercise self-control and forego small wants in favor of strengthening character and building energy. A dharmic yogi can achieve anything in this world. Food, material necessities, and wealth come of their own accord only to be followed by the knock of fame at the door. Such a yogi welcomes these things but stays true to their quest for Atman, the great power that runs the universe.

BE A DISCERNING STUDENT

Religious teachings often depict life as a battle of good and evil in which morality on earth is rewarded in the afterlife. Yoga offers an alternate view in which the choice to act morally is the first of many steps toward realizing our full human potential here and now. Some yoga schools draw a distinction between relative and absolute morality. Relative morality includes all the attitudes, understandings, behavioral norms, and ethical principles that help create a safe, equitable, and humane society. SK spoke of relative reality as the domain of dharma, which he associated with the first three aims of life. All relative moral questions can be resolved by returning to dharma's foremost principle of ahimsa or non-harming. To cause suffering is wrong, and to alleviate suffering is right.

Where dharma clarifies our right relationship to society, absolute morality concerns our relationship to the whole of the cosmos. Its importance only becomes evident after an ardent yogi has embarked on a quest to realize the deeper truths of life. SK called this *the realm of moksha*, and any moral questions regarding it can be resolved by returning to a different foremost principle that can help guide your meditations. Whatever brings you more closely in touch with your essential self and into union with ultimate reality is right, and whatever dims your connection to them is wrong.

I have no reservations in crediting the dharmic teachings of SK for helping me live a good life. But I do not believe they guarantee success. Real life is not a morality play in which villains are punished and the righteous sooner or later always get rewarded. Many of my colleagues at Kripalu Center were high minded and ethical. To me they seemed in all ways deserving. Yet not all of them met with success, and a few encountered tragic setbacks. It seems that all any of us can do is courageously conduct the experiment of yoga while knowing the results are outside of our control.

APPLYING THIS CHAPTER IN PRACTICE

Swami Kripalu spent his first decade as a monk intensively practicing character building. Reflecting on his life, he described this as the period in which he moved through the first two limbs of yoga: yama and niyama. The single-minded practice of character building instilled his life as a young swami with passion and purpose. Some years later, it brought him fulfillment and fame. That prepared him to begin his secluded practice of asana, pranayama, and meditation in mid-life, which he took up with equal intensity in an ardent quest to scale the ladder of yoga to its highest rung.

It is important to note that this bifurcated path that SK walked is not the approach he recommended for others. He taught an integrated path of yoga in which postures, pranayama, and meditation were practiced right from the outset to reinvigorate the body and mind. Yet he continued to emphasize the importance of yama (morality) and niyama (ethics), instructing new students to anchor themselves in the process of character building and learn the principles of karma yoga soon after commencing their on-the-mat practice.

Personally, I've found the practice of character building more of a traveling companion than a preliminary stage of yoga. Even as I write these lines, the process of strengthening my moral backbone continues.

For me, adhering to good conduct has required a lifelong discipline that has lessened some in intensity but never fully relented. That framed list of the restraints and observances still hangs in our yoga room, and I continue to look at it every morning.

To read a teaching story illustrating the foundational role that dharma and character building are meant to play in the practice of yoga, see "The Tax Collector and the Mahatma" in Appendix 2.

As individuals we are all continuously desiring; it is important not to forget or deny that fact. These desires will create disturbance everywhere unless we pursue them properly, which is why the scriptures say, "Whatever you desire, obtain it according to dharma." Money is a useful tool in buying different commodities; even swamis have a need for it. It is important to earn it honestly. People also have a need to contribute to their communities and be recognized by their peers. They desire status and respect. Eventually a person will want nothing back from society. They simply desire to serve. A yogi grows beyond even this need and arrives at the place where they want only to end this friction that creates a continuous disturbance in the mind. This is the desire for moksha.

CHAPTER 8

SANATANA DHARMA: A YOGA-BASED LIFE PATH

The spiritual path that I teach is called Sanatana Dharma. As practiced by the rishis of ancient India, Sanatana Dharma is not a sectarian religion. It is the performance of skillful actions that lead to the direct realization of truth.

After sorting out all the generic ways that Swami Kripalu used the word dharma, it became easier for me to understand one specific usage that played a prominent role in his teachings. *Sanatana Dharma* was SK's name for the entirety of the yoga-based wisdom tradition developed by the Indian sages. The word *sanatana* means eternal and unchanging. In this context, dharma has two distinct meanings. The first is truth, making Sanatana Dharma the eternal truth.[1] The second meaning is path, making Sanatana Dharma the unchanging path to realize this truth.

If there is an absolute truth underlying the relative surface of reality, it must be integral to existence, operating like the natural forces of gravity and magnetism. Immutable forces and the scientific laws explaining them can't be invented. They can only be discovered by abandoning preconceptions, inquiring deeply into how life actually works, and utilizing instruments able to register subtle impressions outside the range of normal awareness. This describes the path of Sanatana Dharma, which

---

[1] The eternal or timeless truth referenced by Sanatana Dharma is synonymous with Brahman. The sages saw everything in material form as relative and in flux. In their view, Brahman alone was absolute and unchanging. Yoga is a synonym of Sanatana Dharma, as it means both the unified field of ultimate reality (Brahman) and the disciplines that enable you to realize it within yourself as atman. These parallel terms point to a singular teaching.

eschews theories in favor of yoga techniques that heighten the human faculties needed to directly apprehend truth.

> *The great yogis discovered the truth of the soul and crafted a way to realize it called Sanatana Dharma. It's a way of living that brings forth the supreme potential of man. The yogis never felt a need to own Sanatana Dharma, so it doesn't have a nationality. They refused to reduce it to a creed, so no one has ever done missionary work for it. I have practiced it for many years and never once thought that it belonged to me or India. That's because followers of this path think of themselves as citizens of the world.*
>
> *The truths of Sanatana Dharma have been realized by the saints and spiritual masters of all times and lands in their meditations and through divine revelation. Truth cannot belong to any one race, religious sect, or nation. It does not recognize such narrow distinctions and makes itself available to the whole world. This truth is like the sun; it bestows light on everyone. Once a seeker has known ultimate truth, his whole life is guided by it. Truth becomes his only guru and his only God.*
>
> *The rishis called Sanatana Dharma the immortal religion because the truth it points to cannot be destroyed. Absolute truth alone is permanent; everything else is transitory. Those who have experienced this truth teach that religion is a science. They see all its different approaches as leading to a common goal: the direct knowing of truth. Meditation and other practices are tools to help us discover truth. As aspirants we must respect truth wherever we find it, because genuine spirituality is not a matter of opinion but a search for the experimentally proven truth. Yoga was born out of this Sanatana Dharma culture.*

SK was careful to distinguish the inquire-to-discover approach of Sanatana Dharma from doctrinal religion.[2] Where creed-based religions often divide the world into opposing factions of believers and

---

[2] The English word religion comes from the Latin root *religare* meaning "that which unites." This parallels one of dharma's oldest definitions: "that which holds together." I am using the term "doctrinal religion" to describe sects that emphasize the acceptance of a creed or codified belief system on faith as the essence of what it means to be religious.

non-believers, Sanatana Dharma invites humankind to unite in a shared search for truth. Like the sages of old, SK saw yoga as a means of cultivating the capacity to find answers to life's deepest questions in the sanctuary of our own hearts and minds. Religiosity has never been a pre-requisite for its practice, as Sanatana Dharma affirms the equal efficacy of theistic and non-theistic approaches. Even though SK was himself a lover of God, he made this point clear to his students:

One individual believes in God. Another is unwilling to accept the existence of anything above nature. These are the two primary opinions in the universe of human thought, and Sanatana Dharma accepts that either stance can serve as the base for spiritual advancement. The authors of the old scriptures were open-minded. They wanted their students to evaluate a system of thought by experimentation and then decide for themselves. There was no disregard for any individual or decision, as all forms of truth and truth-seeking were respected. After studying their founding principles, a person setting out on the path of Sanatana Dharma can choose to practice seshvara (with God) or nareshvara (without God) yoga. While differing on the belief in God, the two are very similar. The gates of Sanatana Dharma are open to all, with everyone able to travel under truth's broad banner.

SK never encouraged his Western followers to become Hindus, yet all the yoga centers and ashrams established by his students outside of India adopted Indian customs and promoted its culture. This was not his approach. Before coming to the United States, he studied a Gujarati translation of the Bible to learn about the religious background of the people he would be meeting. Then, while settling in at the original Kripalu Center in Pennsylvania, he wanted to learn more and was given an English text organized around a set of illustrations depicting the events of the New Testament. Viewing the artwork inspired him to write a moving book on the life of Christ:

Yesterday I received a book that had a picture of holy Christ hanging on the cross with nails in his hands and feet. I was so overwhelmed by his agony that I had to close the book. The picture created a profound change in me, and I was carried into the past two thousand years ago, and the life of Christ came alive. To me, Shri Christ is one of the great light bearers of the world whose teachings illuminate the mystical science known by all the torchbearers of true religion.

In the talks he delivered during his four years in America, SK encouraged interested listeners to integrate yoga practice into their native culture and the religion of their birth. This advice reflects the inclusivity of Sanatana Dharma, which today's theologians would consider an example of "religious pluralism." In our time, there is heightened and rightful concern about cultural appropriation—the insensitive or unfair adoption of the ideas, practices, and meaning-laden elements of one society by members of another and typically dominant society. While proud of India and its rich heritage, it's interesting that SK did not think in these terms, at least in the domain of yoga:

If yoga is really a science, a faithful practitioner from any country or culture should be able to apply its principles and experience its truth. Despite this, the yoga teachers of today encourage their students to adhere to Indian ways. My guru taught me that a yogi is a universal person free from the bondage of country who acts as a well-wisher of the world. I shall teach you yoga from that point of view only. Then you may compare its teachings with the wisdom of your own culture from an independent angle and give it proper justice. Defects are found in everything. Even within yoga, some sects denounce the teachings of other sects. Instead of pointing out defects, Sanatana Dharma instructs us to seize upon the merits of different approaches. I am sure there are many valuable lessons that India can learn from the way things are done in the West.

In the four decades since Swami Kripalu resided at Kripalu Center, two religious trends have pulled American society in opposite directions as shown by a series of studies conducted by the Pew Research Center. First, it's clear the population as a whole is steadily shifting away from organized religion. A decreasing number of people describe themselves as "religiously affiliated" with over one-fifth of all adults now identifying as "spiritual but not religious." Demographers debate the causes of this growing divide between religion and spirituality. Some point to the growing influence of science and a disaffection with churches beset by scandals whose leadership is overly concerned with money, power, and politics. Others draw attention to the mainstream's growing interest in therapeutic tools to foster well-being, which leads many to reject the idea that joining a religious institution is the best way to foster spiritual growth. Whatever its cause, SK's teachings on Sanatana Dharma foreshadowed this trend, which has clearly contributed to yoga's popularity.

The main objective of many religious leaders is material. They are building up the strength of their institution without traveling its path of realization. As a result, they encourage blind faith and take recourse to creeds to enlist followers. This is not the way of Sanatana Dharma, which encourages individual truth-seeking. Where religion says, "Our founder was a great person who brought the truth to light," Sanatana Dharma says, "The greatness of truth brought this particular person into the light." It is this reverence for truth that inspired the venerable sages of the past. When a luminary who has progressed to the highest ministers to the world, the people truly benefit and efficacious pathways of spiritual practice naturally grow up around them.

While many Americans have left the ranks of the religious, a subset of the population has become more devout. This is the second trend noted by the Pew Research Center, which reports that these individuals often self-identify as "evangelicals." The term evangelical comes from a Greek word for "good news" (*euangelion*), which originally referred to any assembly subscribing to basic Christian values. In post-colonial America, the term became synonymous with revivalism, a Christian movement led by fiery preachers intent on persuading outsiders to adopt its particular beliefs. SK spoke to the dangers of this kind of thinking:

Truly religious people are naturally humble and tolerant. Having placed themselves beneath a higher power, they are eager to serve and receive knowledge from everyone. If a self-righteous person becomes a religious teacher, they presume to know more than they actually do. Having fallen in the trap of pretentiousness, they misguide their disciples. Real religion always creates unity among diverse peoples. If the teacher you are following is sowing division, they are only propagating the illusion of religion.

While calling out the shortfalls of organized religions, Swami Kripalu did not take a secular stance. He believed that something akin to religious earnestness was an essential ingredient of the yoga taught by its founding sages. But it wasn't necessary to adopt or feign a pious attitude, as an authentic spark of spiritual inquiry would be kindled by the practice itself, regardless of whether the practitioner was a theist, atheist, or agnostic.

There are good reasons why some people believe in God, and others accept only material existence, arising from their different backgrounds and life experiences. That is why in Sanatana Dharma the practice of yoga is always coupled with a question. Who am I? What am I? Who is God? What is this whole universe about, and where did it come from? At some point in practice, a genuine question like this will emerge directly from the intuition or reasoning of the individual, and not through the encouragement or influence of anyone outside. The answer to this question cannot be found in books. For that, one has to enter into the body, draw close to the soul, and receive inner guidance.

When this inquiry ignites, an aspirant grows hungry for truth. But a doorway to the truth will not open unless appropriate investigations are made into the nature of the self, God, or the universe. That is why a special type of faith is needed by all aspirants for their practice to be successful. They must have faith that a human being can experience the truth to which all such questions point. If an individual's faith in the approach of yoga is strong, it will inspire actions that take them away from mental conceptions and toward the truth.

The eternal truth of Sanatana Dharma can never be known by the mind because it is beyond all ideas and notions. Truth realization only becomes possible when the agitated, extroverted mind is transformed into a steady, introspective mind. Only then are the conditions right for us to step outside the mind and all its filters to see what is truth and what is falsehood. This is a real way to reach to the highest. Whenever it occurs, anyone of any disposition experiences one and the same ultimate reality.

SK knew that relatively few Americans come to yoga seeking an alternative religion. Most are looking for health, stress-relief, and a way to experience greater peace of mind. He considered these laudable goals and wanted all of his students to achieve and enjoy them. Yet he also knew that right thinking alone does not empower; nor do calisthenics transform. In order to be truly transformative, yoga has to bring a person into unmediated contact with their spiritual source, and progressively deepen that direct connection over time.

While encouraging individuals to take up the practice of yoga in whatever way works for them, Swami Kripalu didn't shrink from saying that a yoga student intent on self-actualization and Self-realization must undertake its practice with a purposeful zeal on par with that of religious adherents. That's why the Sanatana Dharma he taught is more than a cogent philosophy coupled with a beneficial set of physical and mental exercises. It is a spiritually-potent wisdom tradition designed to unleash the power of the Self and fuel a life-changing process of spiritual awakening.

An able person can successfully undertake several vocations in life. This is why I encourage my students to stay in society, honoring dharma while also doing spiritual practice. But anyone who wants to travel the path of yoga must make it one of their cherished vocations. It cannot be treated as a casual matter. To create a garland, different flowers are braided together on a single string. To sanctify our life, all our actions must be tied to the thread of spirituality.

There is one other thing a householder yogi must understand. In daily life, we are accustomed to doing several actions at the same time. We divide the mind, which enables us to efficiently attend to different matters. Yet to progress in yoga, we have to unify the mind by channeling all our energy in one direction. This is why there is a twofold practice for yogis living in society. In daily life, we employ the mind as needed to skillfully discharge our duties. But in the meditation room, we must give up all the distractions of the world and feel as if we are sacrificing our whole life to a holy cause. An adept traveler on this twofold path learns to close the gates of the senses to all outer activities and keep the mind's entranceway open only to the Truth. This one-pointed meditation steadily leads them toward a yoga (state of unity consciousness) whose final attainment is never the result of one's effort and concentration. It is always experienced as grace.

BE A DISCERNING STUDENT

It's a bit ironic that the term Sanatana Dharma does not appear in the Vedas, Upanishads, or other traditional texts.[3] The name was coined by the leaders of the Indian independence movement in the late nineteenth century as an alternative to Hinduism. Hindu is a Persian word that originally meant "those who live on the other side of the Indus River." It was a geographic reference without any religious significance until it was coopted by the colonizing British, who used it to distinguish between members of India's majority religion and Buddhist, Christian, Islamic, Jain, and Sikh minorities.

More than a name, Sanatana Dharma was a new conception of Indian history designed to unseat the paternalistic British Raj, which used India's religious diversity to foment dissension between its different sects and remain in power. The British looked down upon Hinduism as primitive, mired in superstition, and rooted in an outdated caste system. Where Hindu was a pejorative label projected onto them by foreigners,

---

[3] The words sanatana dharma do appear in Section 4-138 of the Laws of Manu, but in an entirely different context: "Let a person say what is true; let him say what is pleasing; let him utter no disagreeable truth; and let him utter no agreeable falsehood. That is the sanatana dharma (eternal law)." The Bhagavad Gita refers to Shaswat Dharma, which means "the truth that comes straight down from heaven." Historians suggest the organizing ideas and perhaps the term Sanatana Dharma itself originated in the 1880s with the Brahmo Samaj and Arya Samaj, two influential religious reform movements that had political objectives. The earliest English usage of Sanatana Dharma as a synonym for Hinduism that I could find was in a speech delivered on May 30, 1909, by the freedom fighter Aurobindo Ghose upon his release from a year of solitary confinement for advocating Indian independence. After prison, Aurobindo left politics and spent the rest of his life developing a modernized approach to the spiritual life he called Integral Yoga. In 1921, Mahatma Gandhi would declare, "I call myself a Sanatani Hindu, because I believe in the Vedas, the Upanishads, the Puranas, and all that goes by the name of Hindu scripture."

Sanatana Dharma was a dignified name in the native tongue designed to foster national pride and inspire interfaith cooperation in opposing colonial rule.

The doctrine of Sanatana Dharma was a bold proclamation that all Indians (including Buddhists, Jains, and Sikhs) share the glorious heritage of its Vedic rishis and Upanishadic sages who realized the eternal truth and established a foundation for Indian civilization that was divinely inspired, spiritually-advanced, monotheistic, and scientific in its outlook. Yoga was central to this doctrine, as each of India's religions was seen to reflect a different facet of a single eternal truth knowable to all through the techniques of yoga. A hundred years later, a simple online search of "Sanatana Dharma" shows that the effort to recontextualize Indian religious history was a dramatic success. While Hinduism remains the common name for India's majority religion, Sanatana Dharma has become the dominant narrative of Indian religious history.

Today's scholars would caution us to remember that the actual history of religious movements on the Indian subcontinent is spectacularly complex. Where the view of the British was self-serving, the leaders of the independence movement had their own biases. They were motivated to overlook doctrinal differences and sanitize India's past of superstition and any elements out of step with modern norms to sidestep controversy and dissension. Some historians go so far as to argue that pre-colonial Hinduism was a conglomeration of disparate and competing sects that only became a unified religion when forced to declare its defining principles in the effort to oppose colonial rule. It's interesting that one of the leading figures in reformulating India's diverse strains of religious thought into an intellectually-sound and inspiring Hinduism was Swami Vivekananda, the spiritual luminary widely credited with bringing yoga to America in 1894.[4]

The principles of Sanatana Dharma were born from the practice of yoga, and all its originators were Indian yogis. Today there is world-wide interest in yoga and its enthusiasts like to wear Indian

---

[4] A century after they were written, Swami Vivekananda's treatises on yoga remain relevant and well-worth the attention of contemporary students. Like SK, Vivekananda was a religious pluralist. He often repeated the Sanskrit credo "sarva dharma sambhava," which means "all religious are equally worthy of respect."

dress, take Sanskrit names, and live in an Indian style. But none of these things show that they understand Sanatana Dharma and its approach. What the great rishis and sages discovered is how anyone from any culture can use the tools of yoga to attain the four goals of human life: prosperity, enjoyment, purposefulness, and liberation. Sanatana Dharma grants tremendous freedom with regards to life's externals but stays firm on the need for the systematic practice of its principles, which produce the same results in the body and mind of a practitioner from any country. After scientists discovered the principles of electricity, people everywhere started utilizing motors, lights, radios, and televisions. In the same way, the whole world can make use of the principles of Sanatana Dharma. Compared to other religions, Sanatana Dharma places a greater emphasis on the goal of Self-realization. This is because the fulfillment of even a highly accomplished and ethical person will remain incomplete unless they gain access to the supreme-most-truth that bestows eternal peace and bliss. Because Sanatana Dharma accepts the truth of all religions and acknowledges the revelations of their various scriptures, it is important to highlight this one distinctive feature of the Indian religions because it is vital to yoga practice.

CHAPTER 9
SANATANA DHARMA IN PRACTICE

My guru used to warn me. After studying philosophy, it's easy to think you've become wise. While reading about yoga, you may feel you've become enlightened. Never forget that accepting the principles of Sanatana Dharma is not the same as direct knowledge of the truth itself, which is only obtained through practice and personal experience.

You might imagine the way to apply Sanatana Dharma in your life is to adopt its principles as a guiding ideology. That's what I did, and looking back it served as a first step. But I couldn't stop there because all of Swami Kripalu's talks and writings reiterated a singular point he considered of paramount importance. Sanatana Dharma is a path of action, and progress along that path is only made through practice.

Sanatana Dharma teaches that everyone has equal claim to yoga and its benefits. But everyone must also observe a cardinal rule, which is to engage in regular practice. Without practice, even an ordinary task cannot be accomplished. The same principle applies to yoga, through which extraordinary benefits are possible. By hearing the teachings, an understanding of the path may be gained, but remember that success does not come in that way. Success comes only through the repeated practice of yoga techniques.

SK often described Sanatana Dharma as a linked network of yoga-based pathways that traverse a tall mountain and ultimately lead to a single summit.[1] Of course this was only a metaphor. The spiritual path is not a route to a destination. It's a course of action designed to produce a definite and desirable set of results. Yet those actions, when properly taken, spark a developmental process that feels like it's taking you somewhere. Throughout his teachings, SK shed light on the twists, turns, and defining milestones of this metaphorical journey, and his granular guidance on the path of yoga pervades this book. This chapter conveys his big-picture perspective on the spiritual path as encoded in the symbolic stories he told of people navigating its critical junctures.

Once a student understands that yoga is a tool to bring forth the full power of the self, SK's advice was to get started on the journey by commencing some practice without delay. He didn't prescribe any particular regimen. He considered the technique selected as secondary to making the crucial shift from theory into action. Whatever practice is undertaken, it should be carried out for an amount of time that enables it to bear fruit. One person might sign up for an instructional series of yoga classes. Another might commit to meditating fifteen minutes every morning for a month. A third might cut all junk food out of their diet for a week. He packaged his advice on this entry-level practice in a whimsical tale called "The Farmer's Vow" that appears below in Appendix 2. The symbolism of this teaching story only becomes apparent when the reader discerns its message on the importance of putting theory into practice.

> *To read uplifting books or listen to spiritual discourses is good, but to practice even a little is of the utmost importance. Real knowledge is obtained only through personal experience, and for experience practice is indispensable. The day you start to practice, your true progress will begin.*

Why should a new student leap right into practice? SK was confident that anyone who put yoga to the test would taste its benefits. And this would inspire them to study it more closely to gain the conceptual

---

[1] The yogic path is meant to transport a practitioner to liberation or moksha. The Greek sages spoke of a similar ultimate destination they called *telos*. Aristotle believed that human beings can find telos/purpose in life by gaining metaphysical knowledge through the disciplines of philosophy. SK taught it can be reached by pursuing dharma and attaining *vidya* (direct spiritual knowledge) through the disciplines of yoga. Once again, these are parallel terms pointing to a single truth.

overview needed to support a systematic practice. A key element of this overview is an accurate conception of the yoga tradition. Many people come to yoga with the mistaken belief that it's a single, homogeneous spiritual path. In actuality, there are many different yoga schools, each offering a distinctive way up the mountain. Students who lack this understanding inevitably become confused as they encounter contradictory teachings and signposts pointing in different directions. Edified by this knowledge, a student can enter a second phase of yoga practice during which they sample a variety of approaches.

> *Here it is necessary to remind a student that many paths of yoga are available in this world. While their practice leads to a singular truth, individuals are of different natures and each must find their way onto an appropriate path leading to it. In ancient times, the forest-dwelling sages were complete teachers. Having reached yoga's peak, they could see how all its pathways ascend to that highest place. When accepting a student, they were able to determine exactly where that student was coming from and direct them accordingly. Today only incomplete teachers are available who teach from their experience in following a particular path to a preliminary point. Given this fact, what is a newcomer on the path of yoga to do?*
>
> *At first, teachers may be numerous. The role of these teachers is to impart general knowledge to help us commence our journey. As students, we must understand that great yogis of the past discovered a diversity of yogic paths to enable us to move in the direction of happiness. Some of these lead to health and peace of mind, others to fulfilling desires, still others to obtaining various powers, and a few all the way to everlasting bliss. Contact with teachers who represent these different approaches enables us to find a view that we earnestly believe to be true and a path that we feel inspired to walk.*

Many benefits come from this period of exploratory practice, which can remain fruitful for years. Many readers are likely in this stage; life explorers perusing this book to enhance their general understanding of spirituality and yoga. SK believed that an open invitation to sample different approaches would eventually lead a student to pick one path and pursue it ardently. When this occurs, it is an important milestone in the life of a yogi, and one likely to herald a significant shift in their practice, especially if it involves working with a teacher. That's because each path defines its goals differently and uses the tools of yoga in distinctive ways to accomplish them. These subtle differences must be understood and honored for the practices to produce their promised results.

> *Everyone understands how the same journey can be made in an automobile, boat, or airplane. In a similar way, the various yoga paths are different vehicles to speedily make the journey to the Self. Choose your path carefully, for you will only be able to keep up your practice if you have tremendous faith and interest in it. Once this choice is made, a whole set of different values come into play. Steep yourself in the literature pertaining to your path. Study the lives of its saints and masters. Keep contact with its respected teachers. To get water you have to dig vertically, at times through hard ground and rock, until you have a deep well. If you wander horizontally, you will dig only shallow holes and never strike water. This is why it is said that a seeker's path to Self-realization can only be one.*
>
> *Today many people are hungry for spiritual growth. In search of gurus, they go from ashram to ashram. They read one scripture this week, and another the next, all the while dabbling in different techniques. This spiritual restlessness is not the way to success. Here is how to become stable in your yoga practice. First you must intelligently examine all the different approaches. Then select the one that is convincing, that feels as if belongs to you, even if it is not attractive to others. A good student is one who can be calm and patient while searching out their path.*
>
> *If you go from approach to approach, you will collect a storehouse of conflicting advice and your mind will grow confused. If you take a single path, holding fast to its founding principles and refusing to give up on your practice of its techniques, your mind will become steady and eventually grow still. Only then can you realize that spiritual knowledge seems to come to us from contact with some person or path, but that is not really true. All spiritual knowledge arises from the atman or soul, whose very nature is illuminating,*

> *and not from anything or anyone outside of us. The purpose of an established path is to help us persist in our practice and remove the layers of ignorance that block the emergence of this self-knowledge.*

I was poised on the precipice of this stage when I met Swami Kripalu in 1981. I'd started practicing yoga postures as physical exercise in high school. During college my interest in spirituality was kindled. I surveyed the world religions, sampled different styles of meditation, and participated in many of the consciousness-raising movements prevalent in the 1970s. Standing on the threshold of adulthood, I was actively seeking a yoga-based path of self-development.

After reading *Autobiography of a Yogi*, I joined the Self-Realization Fellowship and signed up for its correspondence course. I'd completed a year of weekly lessons, and was eligible to be initiated onto its path of Kriya Yoga, but something held me back from making that commitment. At the time, I felt hesitant because there was no active teacher or practitioner's community in my area. Looking back, I had not yet found the one path that most resonated with me. After meeting Swami Kripalu, the question of what teacher to follow was answered, and from that day forward my spiritual life orbited around his teachings, and the pace of my progress picked up.

SK reverenced yoga's rich mix of teaching lineages for preserving the hard-earned wisdom of all the sages who'd walked their diverse pathways to spiritual awakening. One element common to all of these lineages is the role of systematic practice, which is also recognized as essential to transformative learning by a new branch of psychology called the science of expertise. Pioneers in that field have coined the term "deliberate practice" for the gold-standard learning method proven to produce world class athletes, virtuoso musicians, international chess champions, and top-tier brain surgeons.

According to psychologist Anders Ericsson, a practice is deliberate if its techniques are done with a guiding purpose in pursuit of clearly-defined goals.[2] Instead of repeated attempts conducted with a vague expectation of improving overall performance, deliberate practice is a structured training in which practitioners accomplish a series of

---

[2] Anders Ericcson and Robert Pool, *Peak: Secrets from the New Science of Expertise* (Houghton Mifflin Harcourt, 2016).

targeted steps that together add up to superior expertise. This requires the involvement of an expert teacher or coach able to pass on acquired knowledge and provide feedback on the best way to do things.

The teacher's first task is to ensure that a student properly masters the fundamental techniques, as this provides a firm foundation upon which a superstructure of advanced skills can be built. Next the teacher helps the student develop an evolving set of "mental representations," as superior performance in any field is always undergirded by a growing cognitive sophistication.[3] The ability to actively engage the mind in the nuances of practice is one secret to keeping it alive and life enhancing, as Ericsson notes that repetitive routines are likely to become rote and even deadening. Then performance measures are identified, which enable students to monitor their own progress, spot mistakes, adjust accordingly, and eventually graduate into proficient self-reliance. When all these elements come together, a student not only knows where he or she is going, but exactly how to get there.

It is best to have an acharya (authoritative teacher) who can induct you in the theory and practice of your chosen path. If necessary, this general knowledge can be gained through books. This guidance must not be only heard once. It must be understood in its particularity, which will require you to reflect upon it again and again. Afterwards, techniques like prayer, mantra, postures, pranayama, and meditation can be practiced accordingly. If done properly, these properly-done techniques will bring results.

Ericsson is adamant that deliberate practice does more than enable a student to actualize their inborn potential. It draws upon the adaptability of the body and plasticity of the brain to create entirely new capacities, enabling people to do things that were previously not possible. While proven in its ability to produce Olympians and virtuosos in all fields, deliberate practice is not easy. It demands heightened attention, an ability to sustain times of near-maximal effort, and the motivation

---

[3] In yoga, these mental representations are the traditional philosophies, metaphysical models, instructional protocols, and teaching stories meant to inform practice. Performance measures include the various stages of growth and states of consciousness delineated in the texts and teachings.

to consistently get out of one's comfort zone in the quest to uplevel performance.[4]

Neither SK nor the sages upon whose shoulders he stood were trained in the rigorous methods of today's research psychologists. It would be hyperbole to claim the yoga tradition contains all the elements of Ericsson's "deliberate practice." However, it is noteworthy how many of these elements do appear in the teaching story "The Sculptor and His Son" that appears in Appendix 2. In this touching tale, SK likens the process of being trained in a yoga lineage to growing up under the care of a loving father who is both a fine artist and an expert teacher. Gaining skill in the techniques of sculpting is only one facet of a broader growth process that emphasizes character development. As his training nears completion, the young sculptor must find a way to graduate from his time of tutelage into the independence of adulthood and a next phase of artistry that marks spiritual maturity.

A student embarking on a clearly-articulated yoga path should feel confident they have found a trustworthy source of guidance in the quest to accomplish the purposes motivating their practice. There is truth underlying this sentiment, as the consistent performance of an integrated set of yogic teachings can bring many life goals into reach. In return, a student should expect to spend several years learning the ins and outs of their chosen path in the process of becoming an able practitioner. Then comes another period in which a seasoned student grows increasingly inner directed. While continuing to follow the general path set out by their teachers, these seasoned students must individuate and find ways to embody its guiding principles in a life expression that is natural to them. Eventually a dedicated practitioner who has followed their chosen path as far as it can take them confronts a deep truth. Walking an established path can only take you to its end point.

While praising discipleship and the power of systematic practice, Swami Kripalu never lost sight of the fact that the end goal of an established path is to position a practitioner to discover their unique route to realization. Entry into this final phase of the journey can only come from a revelatory inner vision that he called *darshana*.

---

[4] As to the role of effort in yoga, Patanjali states that a student's pace of progress depends upon whether their practice is mild, medium, or intense, with swift success coming to a student whose practice is intensively focused. See Sutras 1.21-22.

The life principles taught by the sages are absorbed gradually through study, experimentation, and systematic practice. Learning these principles requires setting out on a path established by a great guru, because without its methods the mind does not become steady. It can be said the absorption process has four levels. The gross level of a principle is gained by study. Its subtle level is grasped intellectually in contemplation. Its subtlest level arises in thought-free meditation. A practitioner cannot experience the final level—the esoteric truth of any single principle—until reaching its root and experiencing darshana.

Darshana is a glimpse of direct knowledge. Whenever darshana occurs, a vision of the unswerving path leading to the ultimate goal of yoga is obtained. Where the path to a steady mind is a gift of the gurus, the path beyond mind is the grace of God. It is only this revealed path that can lead an accomplished practitioner to the realization of the supreme principle (Brahman) that lies at the core of Sanatana Dharma.

When a practitioner is blessed with darshana, their path has been illuminated with the light of direct knowledge. They need not fear losing their way, even if the territory ahead appears strewn with obstacles.

Shortly after arriving in America, SK spent an entire afternoon recounting the life of the Buddha. It's an epic story, and one he told with considerable flair, but he failed to provide any explanation of why he was telling it. Reading and rereading the transcript, I was determined to discern his intended purpose in narrating this tale in such detail. I knew he considered Buddha one of the world's great yogic sages. Eventually it dawned on me that Buddha's life encapsulates the entire path of yoga, enabling SK to trace the journey of an ardent truth seeker who sets out as a novice, apprentices himself to a series of gurus, courageously embarks upon his own path to attain enlightenment, and goes on to become a masterful teacher, all in a single teaching story. To read "The Life of Lord Buddha," see Appendix 2.

Yoga is a science, but it is a mystical science. We can pursue it only through walking in the right paths shown by venerable ones

> *like Lord Buddha. Coal can be found in abundance but diamonds that give light to the entire world are few. Only through self-discipline, zealous practice, and divine grace does a yogi realize the absolute truth. Such a yogi becomes a powerful teacher because the dharma (path) he teaches is based on his direct and completely true experience. This dharma is an excellent gift back to yoga, as it provides other aspirants the truth-based guidance they need to embark upon their paths. Illustrious souls like Lord Buddha performed penance for many years to become true lightbearers. Many secrets are unfolded by the continuous study of their teachings. You will ultimately find your own image reflected in them, but only if you also perform the penance of practice.*

Today, with yoga's physical benefits touted so prominently, SK's teachings are a reminder that its practice was designed to spark a profound, life-transforming journey. While most of today's practitioners start out seeking health and fitness, there is a message for everyone in the ideas Swami Kripalu puts forth in this chapter. Don't get sidetracked by yoga's social glitz, as its real benefits come from time spent doing the practices. It's okay to try different paths on for size. If one of them calls to you, be willing to commit and see where it takes you. Make no mistake, perseverance is required to go the distance in your practice. If and when the blazes on the trees disappear, remember that disciplined efforts can only take you so far. Open to grace to glimpse your unique way forward.

Yoga was a trek up a mountain to Swami Kripalu, and the distinctive trail he blazed was meant to lead all his students through the broad contours and defining junctures of the path described in this chapter to the base camp of good health and effective functioning. For those wanting to go further, he equipped them with the deep understanding of the eight stages of yoga presented in the next book in this series, enabling them to proceed to the summit of spiritual awakening. But few people come to yoga today looking for a spiritual path to organize their life around. They are seeking the immediate and practical benefits detailed in the next chapter.

> *Any yogi who ascends to the highest through practicing a particular method of yoga comes to know that all its pathways lead to*

the same place. Yet that yogi also knows from experience that each newcomer yogi must begin their ascent by adopting one of these established methods. Imagine a flag on the top of a temple located on the peak of a tall mountain. That flag is constantly fluttering, which symbolizes the agitated state of the mind. An aspiring yogi who wants to satisfy their spiritual hunger and know peace must climb all the way to the mountain top and enter the temple. Even though the act of climbing is part of our nature, making an ascent of this kind requires nothing less than the complete willingness to follow an established path until the fluttering flag comes into sight. Once in the shelter of the temple, the yogi can steady that flag by becoming still inside. But even this pristine stillness is not the ultimate attainment of yoga. That revelation must descend as grace.

CHAPTER 10
HOW YOGA WORKS

Any confusion as to how yoga works should be removed by a proper understanding and application of its scientific principles. Only a false teacher would encourage blind faith. As a yogi, I do not believe in lore or superstition. I subscribe to the experimental method and make it a point to always test things for myself before accepting them as facts.

In his youth, Swami Kripalu wanted to understand how yoga works in rational terms. He turned away from teachers who resorted to magical thinking and references to the supernatural to explain its efficacy. Even after becoming the student of a scientifically-minded guru, he continued to display this discerning disposition. It was a trait he exhibited right up to his death, and one that he felt served him well.

As a teacher, he encouraged his students to be inquisitive and independently-minded, and I took this guidance to heart. After reading about the broad spectrum of goals covered by the Four Aims of Life, I began to wonder: "It makes sense that yoga can improve health and hone self-awareness, but how can its practice reliably produce an all-around success in life?"

Asking and answering this question for yourself is critically important, as each student's understanding of how yoga works, whether clear or murky, informs their time on the mat and establishes the scale of benefits it can deliver. This chapter examines the four reasons known to motivate most people to practice yoga: health and fitness; self-development; peak performance; and spirituality. It sets aside Sanskrit terms and metaphysics to summarize SK's no-nonsense perspective on how yoga works in terms of these practical goals. The model that results is easy to grasp and put to the test in your own life:

> *You may wonder how yoga works or doubt its power. By what means can the promised benefits come from just repeating certain exercises over and over? The way yoga works is mysterious and a full understanding comes only by experience and not by logic alone. Briefly, it can be said that yoga strengthens the body and mind by increasing energy and decreasing scattered thoughts. The vitality, clarity of purpose, ability to concentrate, and boost in willpower that results help you attain the first three goals of life—good character, prosperity, and enjoyment—all the while awakening within a dedicated practitioner their slumbering desire for higher spiritual knowledge.*

HEALTH AND FITNESS

Most people come to yoga to enhance their health. Many want the mix of strength, flexibility, coordination, and respiratory function that adds up to physical fitness. Others seek a refuge from the chronic stress that upsets digestion, disturbs sleep, and often leaves us feeling exhausted by life's unending parade of demands, deadlines, and challenges. Swami Kripalu welcomed all brands of health enthusiasts into his circle of students, as he believed the first task of every yogi is to establish a lifestyle supportive of health and healing.

> *The ancient texts describe the type of person who can practice yoga successfully. An aspirant may be weak, diseased, aged, or even senile. All are eligible to practice if they are willing to work at it with enthusiasm. For years devotees have consulted me about their physical difficulties, and I have tried to help them find appropriate remedies. Some have found health by changing their diet. Others by doing asanas or pranayama. Some by meditation, and still others by combining yoga with modern medicine. In my experience, yoga provides an overarching approach to healing in which even late-stage diseases can be treated and often cured.*

SK might have explained yoga's ability to uplift health by asking you to imagine an Indian farmer like many he knew in the Narmada River valley where he lived. Circling a deep well dug at the center of his field, the farmer's ox draws water from the ground. Diverting this water through a series of open irrigation ditches, he waters one plot, and then the next. By carefully cultivating his crops in this manner, the farmer prospers.

A yogi nurtures the body in much the same way. Connected to the wellspring of his spiritual source, rhythmic breathing draws abundant energy into the system. Performing one posture after another, the yogi releases tension and blocks, channeling revitalizing energy to all regions of the body. Resting in relaxation, body and mind are suffused in healing energy. Entering meditation, the energy freed up by these bodily practices is available to bring forth his latent capacities for higher functioning. The yogi leaves his mat and cushion feeling refreshed and ready to resume his duties in life.

Everyone moves their body, breathes in and out, and makes their mind introverted during sleep. These are natural processes that commence at birth and continue until death. Seen in this light, all of us are practicing postures, pranayama, and meditation—only haphazardly. Yoga shows us how to do these practices systematically so our lives become healthy, peaceful, powerful, and prosperous.

For anyone in need of healing, learning how to relax is essential. A relaxed nervous system works efficiently, monitoring any deviation from the delicate homeostasis that underlies healthy functioning and acting swiftly to restore balance. It supports an endocrine system that is finely tuned, producing the precise dosage and mix of hormones needed to regulate organ function. It aids digestion, keeps the immune response strong, and uplevels the body's capacity to heal whatever might be ailing you. All these things happen effortlessly, and happen best, when a person is relaxed. Whenever stress inhibits these or other vital functions, relaxation is the natural antidote.

Yoga includes a set of relaxation techniques designed to help practitioners access a special type of rest called *yoga nidra*. This "yogic sleep" is a twilight state between wakefulness and sleep that quickly renews body and mind. Research has proven that yoga nidra induces the relaxation response, a physiological mechanism known to decrease the heart rate, lower blood pressure, reduce stress chemicals in the bloodstream, and enhance immune response. All these benefits come from increasing the activity of the parasympathetic nervous system, which turns off the fight, fight, or freeze response and turns on the body's healing faculties. Alongside its capacity to soothe a nervous system overwhelmed by stress, deep relaxation is the first step on the yogic path of meditation. It teaches us how to relax the body while the mind remains awake and aware. Later, when this skill is applied in sitting meditation, it makes deeper states of consciousness accessible.

> *Yogic relaxation releases tension from the body and helps remove all the stresses and strains of the mind. A lack of relaxation lies at the root of many diseases, emotional problems, and mental disorders. Consciously practicing relaxation causes a ray of hope to shine in the despairing mind, and through it the body obtains new life and fresh vigor. This art of relaxing the body and mind at will should be learned by everyone.*

The majority of today's yoga practitioners are health and fitness enthusiasts. Decades before approaches like "power yoga" became trendy, Swami Kripalu was aware of all the ways that yoga postures performed with proper breathing can help keep the body firm and fit. He also knew about yoga's ability to maintain joint health, preserve range of motion, and remedy structural injuries. On the practical level needed by most students, he felt that all these biomechanical benefits, along with the biochemical effects noted above, were built right into the classic poses. The best way to gain an understanding of them is to find a qualified instructor and start a regular posture, pranayama, and relaxation practice.

After establishing this practice, the next step on the yogic path of health and wellness is to refine your lifestyle, paying special attention to diet, exercise, sleep, and work/life balance. It's the healing power of combining yoga techniques with healthy lifestyle that SK really touted.

> *The energetic quickening and other benefits of yoga come from doing the techniques properly. Some increase the flow of life energy.*

Others remove the obstacles that block its flow. Due to differences in capacity, some people get fast and full benefit from these techniques, while others receive only partial or delayed benefits. It can generally be said that practitioners who follow the rules of health will get the best effects. But to receive the full benefits of yoga, a person must actively want to grow in wisdom and patiently cultivate a lifestyle supportive of their long-term development. Unless guided by this intention, the techniques ultimately prove of limited worth. No one can practice all of these techniques, but that's okay. Pick the one you find easiest to practice regularly, and do it for your personal growth.

SELF-DEVELOPMENT

Another slice of the yoga community is drawn to the practice as a tool for self-development. They are seeking what SK often called *growth*, which is a gradual unfolding into a full expression of our human potential. The quest for growth touches upon every facet of the self and includes all the physical, mental, emotional, and social factors that enable a person to live a productive and satisfying life. A new academic field of positive psychology has emerged in recent decades to study these and other aspects of what's come to be called "optimal functioning."

In psychology, personal growth is achieved through learning, and more specifically through an increase of self-esteem and the acquisition of positive life skills. While recognizing these factors, yoga places its initial emphasis on catalyzing an energetic quickening that works to revitalize the body, sharpen mental acumen, amplify the capacity to learn, increase empathy, and motivate action. After this revitalization, yoga moves on to teach students a wide array of lifestyle practices, modes of thinking, and other techniques that help them act skillfully in life.

Finding this complex of positive traits in long-term practitioners at significantly higher rates than the normal population, scientists tout yoga's ability to increase "global human functionality." Long before this research, SK saw the virtuous cycle initiated and sustained by regular yoga practice as a trustworthy method of achieving the blend of feeling good in your body, outer accomplishment, and inner fulfillment that he called *success in life*. His faith in the power of yoga came from his own life experience in which prosperity, status, and power seemed to flow to him of their own accord.

Practicing postures and pranayama causes the energy body to bloom, casting light on the inner workings of the mind and body. This leads to self-reflection and eventually one-pointed meditation of the highest quality. The self-understanding that results enables a yogi to reach the pinnacles of success both materially and spiritually.

PEAK PERFORMANCE

Stories abound of athletes doing impossible feats in "the zone," artists entering "flow states" that heighten creative powers, business executives training to function at "peak performance," and patients with life-threatening conditions healing themselves through affirmations and visualization. All signs indicate that each of us possesses extraordinary capacities that typically go unsuspected and thus untapped.

If you practice regularly, you will quickly discover that yoga is a powerful ally in the quest to bring your best self forward in life. Time invested on the mat or cushion does more than relieve stress and maintain a base line of physical health. It pays dividends by stimulating a steady stream of insights that help you adapt and evolve in positive ways. At ease in your body, and with abundant energy at your disposal, you naturally feel good about yourself. Radiating confidence, you have the motivation required to take on challenges large and small. When the need arises to pick up new skills, you can do so easily.

Feeling this way, work becomes an outlet for your creativity, and you derive meaning from overcoming the hurdles that always stand in the way of accomplishing goals and maximizing your contribution to the greater good. At home, yoga heightens the mix of self-awareness and empathy needed to sustain intimate relationships. When times of real hardship and loss arise, as they do for all of us, yoga practitioners display the resilience required to persevere in positive actions, and have tools at their disposal to manage stress. Many aspects of peak performance are only partially the result of on-the-mat practice. To realize them fully, you must also apply the off-the-mat techniques of character building and karma yoga—see chapters 17 and 20.

> *Practicing yoga frees up the vital power and the body becomes radiant. As energy builds, practitioners gain vigor and can develop the skills to progress in any line of work. Along with these specific skills, they acquire enthusiasm, patience, cheerfulness, boldness, and an attractive personality. Moreover, they see how to act in ways that create harmony in their close relationships, and find ways to resolve conflicts that bring forth the humanity of all parties. Through such benefits, they quickly attain to a well-rounded success. Watching this theory in action leads a practitioner to realize that even wealth and fame are best obtained through yoga.*

SPIRITUALITY

Over one third of individuals taking a beginners yoga class report a desire to deepen their spirituality. Exactly what that means is open to interpretation. In contemporary jargon, spirituality is a sweeping term. It's used to refer to a broad spectrum of ideas that includes a belief in an ultimate reality beyond the material universe; engaging in a personal search for meaning and purpose, or a quest to experience the sacred; being committed to living in accord with one's highest values and ideals; and an experiential sense of being connected to something larger than ourselves.

With most classes focused on the physical, it's easy to forget that yoga has always been a way for individuals to connect to the singular power and intelligence that informs all of existence and indwells our being. This is how the yogic sages defined spirituality, which tracks with its original Latin meaning of spirit as the "animating and conscious principle in humans." The use of the word "spirit" in this book is not meant to imply the truth of any religious dogma. It is simply a verbal way to recognize that a deeper dimension exists within everyone that is perpetually fresh and creative, unblemished by life, and brimming with energy. Yoga is designed to bring you into direct contact with this dimension of your being as the manifesting source of your body and mind.

When you become hungry, the desire for food arises automatically. In the same way, when you become hungry for good health, you will run to postures and relaxation. When you become hungry for inner peace and growth, you will run to meditation. This is why the scriptures teach that the body is the first and best means of attaining spirituality. If you practice just a little bit, but every day regularly, your love of health will naturally become an appetite for psychological growth and spiritual awakening.

The experiential reality of spirit is core to the way yoga has traditionally been practiced. To uplift physical health, we must discover spirit as our energetic source and free up the flow of vital energy throughout the body. To stimulate growth and actualize our human potential, we must develop our mind's ability to channel this intelligent energy and utilize it in all areas of our life. In the later stages of yoga, we find that the indwelling spirit is not only a source to draw upon. It's also a portal beyond the limits of the thinking mind that enables us to transcend the confines of our everyday identity to experience what today's scientific researchers call non-ordinary and unitive states.

These experiences show us that there is an ecstasy that is not the result of gratifying the physical senses, fulfilling the goals of the mind, or even making the world a better place. It is an existential joy that emanates directly from the unity of self and spirit, which brings a mental peace that surpasses intellectual understanding. Research is proving that touching into these deeper states of consciousness, even for fleeting moments, infuses meaning into the lives of yoga practitioners and markedly raises their levels of happiness and resilience.

Spirit has a unique quality. It is transpersonal, absolutely the same in you and others, and entirely free of egocentric concerns. Cut off from a vital spiritual connection, we feel separate, isolated, and alienated from our authentic selves. Yogis and sages from all the world's wisdom traditions have taught that this sense of separateness is the root cause of human suffering. As you begin to recognize spirit in yourself, you increasingly see it shining in others, and reflected in the world around you. As the myth of separation falls away, so does suffering.

> *Whether householder or monk, we are constantly confronted by the same problem: separation. Yoga shows us that we are not isolated. We live in a family, in a town, in a country, in a hemisphere, on a planet, in a galaxy, in a universe, and so on. In truth we're connected to everything. A practitioner's direct experience of non-separation is the apex of the yoga I teach, which is profound and worth studying.*

SK saw the desire for depth spirituality in a developmental context in which it arises naturally over the course of a long-term yoga practice. His advice to the majority of us dealing with jobs and family responsibilities was to focus on generating health and growth, allowing the desire for spiritual awakening to assert itself when the time was right.

BE A DISCERNING STUDENT

SK's ascent from poverty and what he called *the sea of insignificance* to the stratosphere of Indian society was meteoric. As his biography makes clear, yoga brought him of all four aims of life in abundance. While drawing inspiration from his life and teachings, don't make too much of his or anyone else's experience. Instead, conduct your own experiment.

> *Yoga practice creates a sanctuary, and it is only by regularly taking refuge in this sanctuary that a practitioner attains the goals of health, worldly success, and spiritual growth. I was very young—only nineteen years old—when I met my guru. Ambitious and thirsty for knowledge, I saw no avenue to attain what I wanted and thus despised my life. He taught me yoga in such a unique way, and I have always tried my best to practice it. Now, all these years later, success has come my way and thousands of people think me to be a great and learned man. I can say without pretense that I am surprised and amazed at what his teachings have wrought in my life. Without them, I could never have reached so far.*

CHAPTER 11
A MAP TO GUIDE YOUR JOURNEY

A map of the world must be drawn on a small piece of paper to be helpful. Knowing this, the great teachers of the past developed diagrams to inform the practice of yoga. A student who learns the secret of the diagram can traverse the yogic path by a very direct route.

After moving into a guru-led ashram, I expected my route to the higher stages of yoga to open up and come clear. True to Swami Kripalu's legacy, the community of 350 residents that Danna and I had joined was committed to practice. Collectively, we were exploring every aspect of yogic living. For a time, it felt exhilarating to ground ourselves in the ashram lifestyle and come up to speed with the group. But a few years into our residency, something else became clear to me. While moving fast, I was not making much forward progress. Truth be told, I was going in circles.

Even within the supportive ashram environment, something essential was lacking in my practice. What I needed was a mental picture that showed where the path was leading and how the techniques of yoga could take me there. At the time, I wanted something simple to hold onto when the stresses and strains of community life were pulling me in different directions. Yet it also had to be accurate enough to be a trustworthy pointer in the right direction. In search of this missing link, I returned to my study of SK's teachings:

When the goal of an aspirant is Self-knowledge, a diagram arrives without invitation. The ancient sages knew it was difficult for aspirants to understand the process of yoga without the experience that comes from having personally traversed its pathway. In these diagrams, they distilled the yogic approach and its different strategies into a compact form. A diagram provides a way to conceptualize yoga that makes its systematic practice possible. In the tradition of the yogis, these diagrams were kept hidden and only revealed to those ready to receive the keys to yoga.

What I found was a map, but the course it charted did not pass through any external territory. It was a diagram of the human person that provided a blueprint for how the tools of yoga could be used to make an inner journey through all its levels of being. The diagram was centuries old and conveyed in archaic language. Only after translating it into contemporary terms, and then drawing it as a visual image, did I see how it could be used as a map. Almost immediately, my practice started moving in the right direction.

Material science seeks to understand the countless objects that comprise the physical universe. Its field of study is immense. Yoga science has devoted its focus to the individual being. This greatly narrows its field of study to the body, senses, thinking mind, intellect, and animating spirit.

Yoga teaches that anything existing in form always finds its energetic source in the formless. This principle explains how a yogi can use the body to gain knowledge of the highest truth. In the whole of creation, there is only one Spirit, which is both the life-giving Atman and the all-pervading Brahman. There is also only one matter, as both the material world and our body belong to the realm of nature.

The yogi who journeys from the gross body through all the subtle layers of mind arrives at the spiritual source from which ensues the creation and sustenance of the universe. Material scientists use instruments like the telescope and microscope to amplify outer awareness and make their discoveries. Similarly, this discovery of the yogis is only made possible by the instruments of asana, pranayama, and meditation, which heighten inner awareness by overcoming external distraction. Seen in this light, the spiritual masters of India and the great scientists of the western world are brothers and sisters belonging to the same family.

THE FIVE SHEATHS OF THE SOUL

One evening I was reading a photocopied translation of SK's then-unpublished commentary on the Hatha Yoga Pradipika when I came upon this section:

In some of the ancient yoga texts, a description is found of the five sheaths of the soul: the sheath of food, the sheath of life energy, the sheath of mind, the sheath of intelligence, and the sheath of bliss. These sheaths indicate the form taken by the formless atman in the causal, subtle, and gross bodies. The purpose of this description is to point out the pure intelligence, splendid glow, and all-pervading spirit that underlies the mind. The bliss of the innermost sheath does not mean delight, as delight and misery are the twofold reflections of mind. When the yogi's meditative experience does not come from the mind or senses, but rather from the soul itself, it is timeless and stable. Just as a person who rests in deep sleep finds their cheerfulness renewed every day, so a yogi who through meditation can rest in the soul becomes always blissful.

This was the first time I'd heard about the five sheaths of the soul. It took a little research in the ashram library to find a section of the Taittiriya Upanishad that matched SK's reference. It describes the human organism as consisting of five *koshas*, or sheaths. The verbatim text is a bit cumbersome but this synopsis captures its essence: From this atman, the sheath consisting of food arose—that is the foundation. Within that foundation, the sheaths consisting of breath, mind, wisdom, and bliss arose to fill it. Verily, it is these sheaths together that have the form of a person.

I was intrigued by the simplicity of this model. In my mind's eye, I pictured five concentric circles with a bull's eye at the center. The outermost sheath is *annamaya kosha*, the sheath made of food, a graphic definition of the physical body. Next is *pranamaya kosha*, the sheath of life energy, which roughly corresponds to the nervous system. Then comes *manomaya kosha*, the sheath made of thought, or the thinking mind. One layer closer to the center is *vijnamaya kosha*, the wisdom sheath that is often called the higher or intuitive mind. The innermost sheath is *anandamaya kosha*, described by the yogis as a field of existential bliss. The center point of our being is not a sheath but a gateway or wormhole into atman, the immaterial soul itself.

As words on a page, the kosha model had captured my interest. To understand it better, I drew a circular diagram:

The Five Sheaths or Koshas

Atman

Bliss Sheath
Wisdom Sheath
Thought Sheath
Life Energy Sheath
Food Sheath

Seeing the concentric circles reminded me of a handout from my yoga teacher training course called The Multi-Dimensional Self. Pulling my manual off the shelf, I was able to find it. While clearly based on the kosha model, it had one glaring omission. At the center of the diagram was the bliss sheath—there was no true self or atman depicted. This ran counter to my reading of the Upanishad and SK's teachings, both of which say that all the layers of our being emerge from a spiritual core. Restoring atman back to its rightful place and relabeling the levels in terms that spoke to me, here is the graphic I ended up with.

The Multidimensional Self

- True Self
- Rapturous Field of Energy/Awareness
- Intuitive Mind and Sublime Emotions
- Thinking Mind and Defensive Emotions
- Nervous System
- Physical Body

As soon as I got this on paper, a series of images flashed through my mind, each a slightly different version of the model. Like the frames of a movie film, they showed how yoga practice is designed to advance a person on the path of self-development. The first image tied each of the major yoga techniques to the primary layer of being it effects. Postures revitalize the outer ring of the physical body. Pranayama activates then steadies the breath, stimulating and calming the nervous system. This combination turns attention inward, making it possible to work effectively with the interior rings. Meditation begins with one-pointed concentration to focus the agitated thinking mind. Meditation deepens as concentrated awareness begins to stream toward the object of contemplation, which brings the insightful intuitive mind online and fosters a range of increasingly subtle flow states that integrate the psyche around the True Self. Meditation culminates in a steady state of unifying presence, which is a precursor to what is always a spontaneous moment of Self-realization.

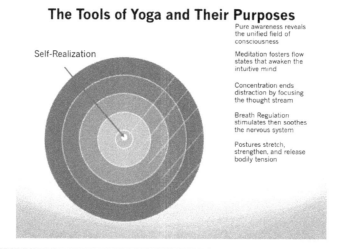

Our manifest being is made up of all the gross and the subtle elements of nature. Truly, it is nothing other than a combination of these elements, which in the end will decay and return to nature. When the gross elements predominate, our awareness is dull and outer directed. When the subtle elements predominate, our awareness is sharp and able to journey within. A thick veil separates the mind and body from the pure and immortal soul or atman. Through the regular practice of yoga, this veil gradually becomes thin. Our awareness goes on developing until the veil is pierced, spiritual knowledge dawns, and the atman is realized.

The next image showed how each technique is a lesson plan in yoga's curriculum of embodied learning. Postures get you out of your head by teaching you to ground awareness in physical sensation. Pranayama activates the breath, amplifying and harmonizing the flow of life energy always moving through the nervous system. Concentration focuses the mind, ending the distracted thinking that keeps you on the surface of your experience. As the mind calms, it feels natural to become absorbed in the soothing flow of inner experiencing. Growing quiet and still inside, you are drawn to rest in the simple state of presence. Having traveled inward to the core of your being, you are poised on the threshold of what could be called enlightened awareness.

Progression of Yoga Experience

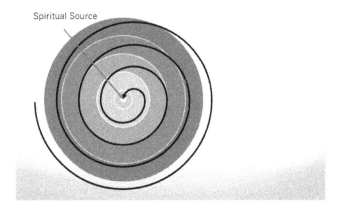

- Resting in pure presence
- Absorbed in the flow states that arise from the intuitive mind
- Concentrated on the details of practice to focus thinking mind
- Attuned to breath and life energy
- Grounded in bodily sensations

Dawning of Enlightened Awareness

Next was a pair of images that shows how this curriculum is pursued in each practice session as a twofold journey. It's first leg is a process of introversion as you apply the tools of yoga to spiral awareness inward through the layers.

Introversion: The Inward Journey to Source

Spiritual Source

After your inward journey completes, you gradually spiral back out in a conscious return to extroverted awareness. The return journey reinvigorates each layer with source energy, empowering you to live more purposefully and effectively. Taking time to facilitate this conscious return is especially important for householders, as it helps avoid a known pitfall. Without it, deep meditation can leave a practitioner feeling that their daily life is bland or even futile, where proper practice produces the opposite result.

Extroversion: The Return Journey Into Life

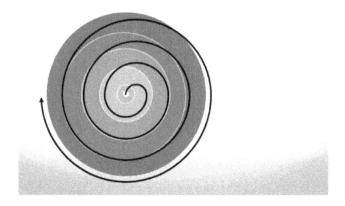

Later, I was amazed to discover that the idea these two images convey dovetails perfectly with the "law of withdrawal and return," a concept that factored prominently into the thinking of Arnold Toynbee, an English historian and philosopher who studied the rise of fall of human civilizations:

> The creative personality undergoes a duality of movement we call withdrawal and return. The withdrawal makes it possible for the personality to realize powers within himself which might have remained dormant if he had not been released for the time being from his social toils and trammels. Such a withdrawal may be a voluntary action on his part or it may be forced upon him by circumstances beyond his control; in either case the withdrawal is an opportunity, and perhaps a necessary condition, for transfiguration. But a transfiguration in solitude can have no purpose, and perhaps even no meaning, except as a prelude to the return of the transfigured personality into the social milieu out of which he had originally come. (from A Study of History)

Accurate knowledge concerning the body, the life energy, the mind, the ego, the individual soul, and the Ultimate Soul is a good friend of the yogic aspirant. Sage Goraksha discusses how this knowledge can be acquired by the systematic practice of introversion. Just as a tortoise draws in its limbs, the yogi turns the mind away from outer objects of perception and toward the Atman. Elsewhere it is said, as the evening sun gradually withdraws its light, the yogi should withdraw attention from the activity of the senses to practice concentration, meditation, and samadhi. Identifying with a superficial and false conception of self is the seed of misery; it matures into a jungle of unhappiness. Identifying with what's true at the core of us is the seed of delight; it matures into a vast garden of happiness. The climax of this happiness is the bliss of samadhi. As soon as an aspirant begins approaching self-knowledge in this way, the spiritual power begins to awaken in them. Their intelligence becomes bright and memory sharp. Creativity blossoms and determination arises to accomplish their goals. Motivations purify until only dedication, service, and the desire to love remain. For one who continues until direct knowledge of the Absolute (Brahman) is gained, the bliss they experience is not momentary but eternal.

While the whole of this curriculum is pursued in each yoga session, there is also a progressive dimension of practice. As you grow increasingly skillful in applying the yogic techniques, you gain easier and swifter access to the innermost layers of your being and the non-ordinary states of consciousness that accompany them. At first these layers are experienced as transient mind states. Over time they become stable character traits, enabling you to periodically make quantum leaps on a journey of self-development. Most people live their entire life from the vantage point of the egocentric self, never suspecting there are higher vistas that only become visible as a person progresses through the developmental stages of this journey. Yoga provides the tools to actualize these intuitively-sensed but seldomly actualized potentials.

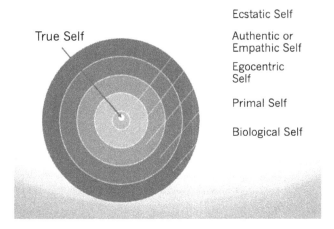

As Swami Kripalu taught:

The self of a beginning yogi and the self of an accomplished yogi are not the same. It is a matter of stages. The starting place of ego is the same for all and reflects an ordinary and often polluted consciousness. The practice of yoga techniques begins to purify the body-mind system. To the extent a practitioner uses those techniques to attain purity of mind, they will discover the self of their pure nature that is bright, imaginative, loving, truthful, and motivated by good intentions. This higher stage of self can easily fall back and be used to acquire all the things wanted by the lower ego, but that will not bring growth, bliss, Self-realization, or even peace of mind. It can be said that the choice to value these higher things marks the real onset of the yogic journey.

The great masters of yoga completed this process, going beyond all the lower stages of self to where true emancipation occurs. Looking back, they explained exactly what those stages are, and noted the qualifications for moving from one to another. Applying this science of yoga, you also can develop stage by stage. If you use the techniques for their intended purpose, the gravitational pull of the ego will gradually subside and your higher potentialities will take over the mind and be actualized. You must remember that the basic tools you are practicing right now have the capacity to take you all the way, if you have the patience to study them closely, understand how they work, and utilize them to attain peace of mind.

THE YOGIC STAGES OF SELF-DEVELOPMENT

- **Biological Self**: The body consisting of its corporeal parts and life-sustaining systems, which like all living organisms has a primitive and largely unconscious sense of self. Thought to be based upon the reptilian brain stem.
- **Primal Self**: Instinctive and quick to respond to a wide range of presenting stimuli. Evolutionary science and Polyvagal Theory suggest mammalian behavior is largely determined by two sides of the autonomic nervous system, its three vagus nerves, and a pre-conscious appraisal of threat and opportunity. Many modern people are disconnected from the kinesthetic intelligence of their primal self.
- **Egocentric Self**: Based on *manas*, or the thinking mind, that combines with the primal self to form the ego of psychology, which yoga calls the ahankara (I-maker). Conditioned, defensive, reactive, clever, opportunistic, transactional, and at times aggressive. Often described as a persona or mask and in spiritual circles is called the "false self." Many spiritual seekers utilize tools from the self-improvement repertoire to cultivate a positive ego with high self-esteem, the ability to relate well with others, valuable life skills, etc. While this is necessary work, it alone will not move you into higher developmental stages. The drive to move beyond the limits of the egocentric self is often what lies beneath the phenomenon psychology recognizes as the midlife crisis. For those practicing yoga, thus developmental shift in identity tends to come easier and earlier.
- **Authentic or Empathic Self**: Based on *buddhi* or intuitive mind and the non-reactive *drishta* or witness. Calm, reflective, creative. In touch with both feeling and

thought. Being much less unconditioned than the ego and grounded in the present moment, the authentic self has a high degree of autonomy and is able to exercise the power of choice. The authentic self is able to express our deeper humanity and the shift to this level is aided by the practice of meditation and witness consciousness, which pull identification out of the thought stream. Relatively few grow beyond the authentic self without the aid of insightful spiritual teachings and practices.

- **Ecstatic or Causal Self**: Based on the yogic conception of the bliss sheath or causal mind. Ecstatic in terms of the original Greek definition that means "the rapture of standing outside your normal sense of self." Spacious, timeless, illumined by the light of what religion would call soul and in touch with what yoga calls the "field of all possibility." The source of existential joy for no reason. Accessed through increasingly subtle flow states and meditative "non-doing."
- **True Self or Non-Self**: Based on the soul or atman or "true nature," which Buddhism describes as empty of form and not personal. Yoga describes it as self-effulgent, which means that it shines with its own light, ineffable, and entirely off the map of normal perception. On the path of yoga, the unity consciousness of samadhi eventually reveals the existence of this true self or non-self.

Yoga is a vehicle to carry us forward. The journey of yoga begins in the land of our lower self and ends in the realm of our highest possibilities. The Sanskrit word "pragati" means to go forward and leave the old behind. To move toward the higher, we have to be willing to leave the old behind. This is what it means to be a traveler on the yogic path of progress.

THE VALUE OF THE KOSHA MODEL

In 2002, I had an experience that cemented my understanding of the kosha model. At the time, I had been on crutches for a year after a synovial tumor destroyed my ankle joint. For months, Danna and I had been searching for a treatment that would preserve my ability to walk, but to no avail. Despite my hobbled condition, I was taking part in the annual Yoga and Buddhism Conference hosted by Stephen Cope. In the opening talk, a visiting teacher was presenting the keystone elements of the Buddhist view. She began with *dukkha*, a term common to yoga and Buddhism, explaining that dukkha is often defined as "suffering" but actually means "a state of dissatisfaction that pervades all aspects of life." Before moving on to explain how the concept of dukkha undergirds the Buddha's Four Noble Truths, she made a seemingly off-hand remark, saying the word literally meant "having a bad axle hole."

For some reason, my mind fixated on that comment. For several minutes the talking head in front of me disappeared as I pondered, "Why would Buddha or any of the yogic sages that preceded him choose that word?" Then I imagined an ox cart rolling along a dusty dirt road. With a bad axle hole, every foot of the journey would be a bumpy ride, something I was viscerally experiencing with my painful ankle and inability to walk. The axle analogy brought to mind the kosha model, which is wheel-shaped. "How," I wondered, "can the practice of yoga or Buddhist meditation fix a bad axle hole?"

I knew that yoga considers *avidya*—not knowing who and what we truly are—to be the foremost of the five afflictions or *kleshas* said to lie at the root of all human suffering.[1] Patanjali makes this point in the Yoga Sutra, and SK often affirmed it in his teachings.

Yoga says the root cause of all our sorrows is avidya—ignorance of our inner self. The stages of yoga practice may be understood as a progression of ways to overcome our natural tendency to identify with the material body and mind, rather than the spiritual atman. To realize atman, we first have to purify the body so we have abundant energy and enthusiasm, but that alone will not liberate us from ignorance. Next, we have to purify the mind, because a clear mind will lead us toward atman, while a dark

---

[1] The Yoga Sutra lists five *kleshas*/afflictions: avidya (ignorance of our true identity), asmita (egoism), raga (the pull of attraction toward objects of pleasure), dvesha (the push of aversion away from objects of pain), and abhinivesha (clinging to life). Each of the last four are caused by the first: ignorance of our true nature. See Sutra II.3.

mind will carry us away from atman. Progressing through these initial stages, the functioning of our intellect is enhanced and we gain the power of discrimination. Only then can we fully engage in svadhyaya or self-study. By discriminating between what we truly are, and what we merely seem to be, our ignorance is dispelled. As self-knowledge dawns, fear and egoism fall away, the push-pull of attraction and aversion subsides, and we are less troubled by wrong actions. This is how yoga unlocks the hidden knowledge of atman and frees us from suffering, but the veiling power of ignorance is vast and not to be treated lightly. It is for this reason that we need many different techniques and stages of practice to gain self-knowledge.

Holding the kosha model in mind, I saw that we all start yoga practice with an egocentric identity coalesced around the thinking mind, which is off-center and not at the hub of the wheel. In other words, our axle hole is out of place. That's why we roughly thump our way through life. To remedy the problem, it's easy to think that you'd just move in towards the center of the circle. But that's not the yogic way. First you must move out to the periphery of the circle, strengthening your connection to the physical body. Anchoring yourself in present-moment bodily sensation is what enables you to break the hypnotism of the thinking mind. Only then can you effectively spiral towards the center, breathing life into each successive layer of your being to regain your sense of wholeness. As you draw close to the hub, you will integrate the body-mind around the true self, a process that unfailingly catalyzes psychological growth and self-actualization. When your axle slots into its rightful place, Self-realization is the inevitable result.

Suppose an aspirant reflects on the scriptures of Vedanta and fully convinced of their truthfulness declares, "I am not the body, life energy, mind, or ego. I am the pure, enlightened, eternal, and emancipated Atman!" While this may be the sincere conclusion of his mental faculty, it is based on indirect knowledge. For this to become his own experience, he must first restore sanctity to the temple of his own body. Then he must to resort to profound meditation.

Only then will it become clear to him that the soul is different from each of its outer sheaths.

The real value of the kosha model is the clarity it brings to on-the-mat practice, which can be summarized in these six steps expressed in the user-friendly language of the ashram's Kripalu Yoga.

- **Come home to your body:** One of the defining characteristics of our time and culture is that we tend to live in our heads, disconnected from the aliveness of the body, and asleep to our deeper self. What yoga calls avidya, psychology calls "self-alienation."
- **Free up the flow of breath:** Deep breathing stimulates cellular respiration, increasing metabolism and uplifting the health of each and every cell. The breath is also intimately tied to the mind and emotions. By regulating the flow and quality of the breath, the emotions can be brought into balance and the mind made calm and clear.
- **Turn on the faculty of feeling:** Focusing your attention inward, you'll encounter a rich mix of sensations and emotions. Instead of pushing them away, invite them to surface as you begin the process of spiraling into source. If you are a trauma survivor, you may need a specially-trained teacher or additional support.
- **Use witness consciousness to enter into flow:** Witness consciousness is the ability to closely observe what is occurring without reactivity or judgment. It is a homecoming to reality, a silent "yes" to the truth of whatever is happening. This ability to simply watch all the distractions that inevitably arise in practice—unproductive or obsessive thinking, self-judgment, blame, comparison, and boredom—is what awakens the intuitive mind and ushers in the flow states that characterize depth meditation.
- **Rest in presence:** As the mind slows down, gaps will appear in the parade of thoughts passing through the foreground of your mind. Use these gaps to sense and see the background field of awareness from which the mind is formed. A good word to describe this matrix of awareness is "presence." Advanced practitioners can use self-inquiry—inwardly asking the question, Who or what am I?—to momentarily stop the mind and touch what lies beyond.

- **Slowly spiral back out with fresh energy and insight for life:** The quality of your inner meditative experience in yoga is vitally important, but the primary purpose of practice is to help you be present and effective in your life. End your practice consciously, which enables you to smoothly transition into action without breaking your connection to source. This helps maintain the quality of your awareness as you get up from your cushion and shift into the off-the-mat practice of daily life.

* * *

I still remember the first time I practiced yoga as a high school sophomore. A hardcover library book lay on the bedroom floor, propped open by the weight of a high-top sneaker. Glancing back and forth from photo to instructions, I was able to page my way through an entire posture series. There were no beginner texts back then, and it was excruciating to bend, twist, and fold myself into the classic poses. I grunted, groaned, and pushed too hard. My alignment was undoubtedly terrible, and the concluding headstand downright dangerous. Yet I knew from the outset that I liked doing yoga, liked the way it made me breathe into the areas of my body being stretched, and especially liked how it left me feeling afterwards. Alongside these first impressions was an intuitive sense that grew stronger as I kept practicing during college. On some level I couldn't understand, yoga was taking me in a direction I wanted to go.

I'm convinced that having the map of the koshas[2] in my pocket is one of the primary reasons I've been able to sustain and deepen my yoga practice over the duration of my adulthood. From the moment I happened upon it, this model worked for me. And as my understanding of it has grown, it's worked even better. Remarkably, all these years later, yoga is still taking me in a direction I want to go.

Suppose you are setting out to drive to a distant and unknown city. First you need a roadmap that shows where it is that you are going.

---

[2] SK also emphasized the usefulness of a second yogic diagram based on the teachings of Tantra. *Swami Kripalu's Ladder of Yoga* presents his teachings on the subtle body and its constellation of energy centers or chakras. While it's clear these two models depict the same territory, they are meant to be applied with different types and in different stages of practice.

From that you can chart a set of directions that describe the stages the journey will take. If you are prepared in this manner, you can confidently set out and begin to make progress. This preparation will not solve all your problems. Enroute you may encounter obstacles. If you get a flat tire, you need to fix it. This is obvious, but you still need to do it. Other obstacles require discernment. You come to an unmarked crossroad in the dark of night. You have to look at your map, think carefully, and choose wisely. Then you have to go forward without knowing if you made the correct turn. Only if you have the ability to bear difficulty and overcome obstacles like these can you eventually enter the city. Making the inner journey of yoga is similar to this, and it is this combination of having a map, doing preparation, and displaying persistence in carrying on despite obstacles that I call "systematic practice."

PART THREE
THE FOUNDATIONAL PRACTICES

After grasping the essential points of yogic science, you must understand that there is a mode of living designed to help your yoga flourish. Eat well and exercise. Cultivate good character and learn to express your love. By observing yourself keenly, create a lifestyle that fosters aliveness in your body and joy in your mind. This is yoga's next step in the overall sequence of human development. If taken, progress in your practice will come easily, and soon you will find yourself standing on the shore of your soul, where the ocean of spiritual knowledge is always roaring.

It is amazing how the yoga tradition stayed vital in India over millennia without the support of any governing body. Instead of a centralized structure, it relied upon the guru/disciple relationship to transmit its teachings from generation to generation.[1] This should not be taken to mean that the tradition lacked rigor. All its major schools had texts and teaching protocols. Before being accepted as a student, an aspirant was required to demonstrate *adhikara*, a defined state of fitness to practice. Desirable qualities had to be displayed, specified behaviors avoided, and various pledges made before instruction in yogic techniques would be given. How different this is from yoga today, where a student pays a class fee and straight away is led in asana, pranayama, and meditation.

You might be surprised to hear that Swami Kripalu, who was a product of a traditional guru/disciple relationship, initially fell short of

---
[1] The Sanskrit term is *guru parampara*, which means "the transmission of a tradition by an unbroken lineage of masters to their adept students."

displaying all of the qualities required to immediately commence yoga practice:

> *Indian gurus have always required fitness on the part of their disciples. My guru only taught me dharma, telling me, "Son, you are not yet ready to approach the highest." But saying this, he also gave me preparatory practices to organize my life that eventually qualified me to practice asana, pranayama, and meditation at a high level. Opinions differ on whether these preliminary practices are rightly seen as part of yoga. Knowing that they were essential for me, I consider them integral elements of the yogic path.*

Exemplary teachers do more than pass on a tradition. They evolve it to a higher level of effectiveness. Seeing the positive role that on-the-mat yoga could play in the lives of novice aspirants, SK guided his students to commence asana, pranayama, and meditation at the outset of their practice. Yet he tried to make sure these techniques were supported by a holistic approach to living that would eventually bring the deeper benefits that yoga is designed to deliver.

> *Unless a person is ready to practice them, yoga techniques will not help all that much. Done mechanically, they may produce temporary benefits, but the type of character development and spiritual growth that I encourage is completely different from the usual health benefits that people associate with yoga. That is why I try to prepare my new students. While they practice asana, pranayama, and meditation, I instruct them to do so within a yogic lifestyle that makes these techniques instruments of their higher growth.*

Chapters 12-20 detail the foundational practices and precepts he considered essential to yoga.

CHAPTER 12
THE SEED DISPOSITION

If you aspire to tread the path of yoga, become the well-wisher of everyone.

The first practice on Swami Kripalu's path of yoga is not a particular diet, posture, breathing exercise, or meditation technique. It's a seed disposition that he called *being the well-wisher of all*. Planted deep in your being, SK taught that this tiny seed of positive sentiment will invariably grow into a great tree of happiness and bear the sweet fruit of success.

While mostly a matter of the heart, there's a logic behind the practice of well-wishing that is important to understand. Yoga invites you to awaken your energy, pursue your soul-purpose, and fulfill all four aims of life. While engaged in this quest, you will circulate in society and interact with others who are also seeking to satisfy their legitimate needs and wants. Yoga teaches that the natural and right relationship between you and these kindred spirits is one of well-wishing. In yogic terms, this is what it means to be a person of true goodwill.

May everyone enjoy good health. May no one suffer from disease. May everyone be blessed. This is the everyday prayer of yogis in India. A yogi knows that when everybody else is prospering they will succeed in their self-efforts and spiritual endeavors too. Anyone can become a well-wisher—whether man or woman, young or old, rich or poor. Well-wishing fosters a pure state of mind that generates good conduct and enables a person to move friction-free in the direction of success and spiritual growth. You

> *can't build the palace of happiness without laying the cornerstone of well-wishing.*

Being a well-wisher is not a moral stance. It's a life-hardy mindset aligned with the way things work. A person who wishes themselves well has the self-esteem required to be upfront about their needs and interests. This directness circumvents the myriad forms of artifice, guilt, shame, and self-sabotaging that all-too-often dulls our internal flow of energy, which in turn stifles health, blocks creativity, and prevents us from acting dynamically. A person who genuinely wishes others well is an attractive partner. They are invested in the welfare of colleagues and willing to sacrifice to support them. A well-wisher's cheerful outlook is contagious, as it's hard to resist the infectious good spirit of someone sincerely focused on fostering the collective good of their team or group.

A well-wisher is naturally collaborative, steering situations toward win-win outcomes, and happy to celebrate everyone's success. When appropriate, a person of yogic goodwill is also able to compete, focusing their energy and skills on achieving a victory free of animosity and enmity. In all these ways, SK taught that well-wishing is a trustworthy vehicle to carry you forward in life.

It would be a mistake to think that well-wishing is an introductory practice meant only for beginning yogis. The most potent and useful yogic techniques are not quick fixes. They are traveling companions and positive traits that must be woven into the fabric of our character and personality. Well-wishing is a discipline commenced at the outset of yoga practice that over time develops into a true yogic attainment. It's also a practice that can be easily applied in your life. The next time you are waiting for a business meeting to start, silently send well-wishes to everyone in the room. After five minutes of well-wishing, check in with yourself to see how the exercise affected you. When the meeting ends, notice if it shifted the way you interacted and performed.

> *A yogi who has reached the stage where the soul becomes one with the supreme spirit is no longer an ordinary person. They feel a deep empathy and affection for others and becomes everyone's friend and helper. Such yogic saints are truly the well-wishers of all. Having lost interest in self-aggrandizement, they silently bestow blessings*

> *upon the deserving and undeserving alike. A seed sown in the ground must grow gradually. In the same way, the seed of true spirituality only matures over time through consistent practice. Do not think that only saints can give blessings. We all affect others and therefore must practice well-wishing to whatever extent we can. You will know you have truly progressed in your yoga when there is no enmity in you for anyone.*

The practice of well-wishing did not originate with Swami Kripalu. The Yoga Sutra says the mind is pacified by adopting a stance of friendliness to others that includes compassion for the suffering, joy for those experiencing good fortune, and dispassion toward the vicious (I-33). The Bhagavad Gita promises that a person relinquishing ill will towards any living being immediately acquires the grace of the Lord (11:55).

SK was being innovative, however, in placing this teaching front and center on his path. He modeled it by always ending his public discourses with the same blessing: *May everyone here be happy. May everyone be healthy. May everyone be prosperous. May no one be the least little bit unhappy at all.* If there is any guidance that can be trusted to hold true at every stage of the yogic journey, it is this inward stance of being the well-wisher of yourself and others. For instructions on how to cultivate this mindset in meditation, see "Becoming the Well-Wisher of All" in Appendix 3.

> *It's impossible to calculate the effect of nurturing just one good feeling in your heart because other good feelings will spontaneously sprout and take root. This practice of well-wishing is like the fabled touchstone that can turn iron into gold because its performance alone can transform an ordinary person into an accomplished individual and ultimately a spiritual master.*

CHAPTER 13
A DISCIPLINE OF DAILY PRACTICE

The profound benefits of yoga are only gained by those who study it through regular practice.

The yoga tradition has long known what neuroscientists are proving through high-tech brain imaging. Ordinary people have extraordinary capacities that can be brought to life by methodical training. The common word for this is practice, and it's a concept central to yoga. Swami Kripalu used a Sanskrit term to explain exactly what the sages meant when they spoke of practice. Abhyasa refers to *a coherent set of yogic techniques that are done regularly, carried on without interruption, for a long time, and conducted with a reverent attitude.*

This type of yoga practice can be contrasted with the popular notion of a workout, an exercise session aimed at physical conditioning. Yoga is designed to deliver a considerably broader spectrum of benefits. Alongside bodily fitness, yoga aims to revitalize the nervous system, foster emotional sensitivity and balance, calm the mind, and spark insights that raise self-awareness. While preserving and expanding current capacities, yoga also gives birth to entirely new and unsuspected possibilities. SK taught that the key to realizing all the good yoga can offer is to establish a regular practice that forges a strong connection between your body, heart, mind, and the energetic source of your being:

By studying the teachings, an intellectual understanding may be gained, but never forget that success in yoga comes only through the repeated practice of its foundational techniques.

He guided students to commence their yoga practice with a simple breathing exercise often called three-part breathing or the complete yogic breath. While the basics of this breath can be learned in a few minutes, it takes a month or more of regular practice to strengthen the respiratory muscles and enliven the neural pathways required to establish yourself in this foundational pranayama technique.

The yoga taught by SK can be described as breath-based because the respiratory capacity gained from this initial period of yogic breathing will carry over into postures and eventually accompany you into meditation. The pranayama he describes below is actually a combination of two traditional techniques. The first is *dirgha* pranayama, with the word dirgha meaning long, slow, and smooth. Making the whisper-like sound at the back of the throat is *ujjayi* pranayama, the victorious breath, which plays an important role in many types of yogic meditation.

Practice dirgha pranayama for one month before beginning postures. In this practice, inhaling and exhaling should be done slowly in such a way that the faint whisper of the breath is audible from the throat region. This whisper-like sound is created by the gentle rubbing of air against the back of the throat. The breath should not be inhaled in haste, or exhaled in haste. Concentrate on letting the in-breath grow long enough to feel as if it is flowing down into the lower belly and all the way up to the upper chest. After inhaling in this manner, it feels natural to relax and let the out-breath completely empty the lungs of stale air. While doing this pranayama, keep the spine straight yet neither tight nor rigid, so the breath can move easily in and out without resistance.

We commence yoga practice with our attention scattered. This leaves our diffused mind easily dragged into divergent currents of thought. Dirgha pranayama proves very useful to overcome this distractedness. Through it the life energy begins to flow through the core of the nervous system versus its periphery, which concentrates the mind. Yoga postures may be started without this preparatory period of pranayama practice. But if yogic breathing is done in advance, the body will be less stiff and the mind more steady, both of which will greatly hasten progress.

After dirgha pranayama has been practiced independently for a month, you need not spend much time on it before doing postures. Taking ten deep breaths at the outset of practice should be enough. An experienced student can also begin with alternate nostril breathing or any variant of skull shining or bellows breath (kapalabhati or bhastrika pranayama). If you want to be victorious in your yoga practice and life, start with dirgha pranayama and learn the art of yogic breathing.

For simple instructions to how to apply these teachings in practice, see "Breathe Your Way into Meditation" in Appendix 3.

SK's guidance on the other aspects of an entry-level yoga practice mirror those of today's teachers. He recommended a balanced sequence of postures done mindfully with proper alignment and rhythmic breathing. The poses should smoothly progress from easier to more difficult, allowing the body to warm up before it is challenged. Practice should end with time for deep relaxation in corpse pose (*shavasana*), which rests the body and renews the mind. He emphasized that all these components must be woven into an integrated practice session, as it's not the deep breathing, active stretching, balanced strengthening, or the moments of relaxed calm that make yoga so effective. It is all of them together.

He believed that it is best for new asana students to work with a skilled teacher in a group setting that enables the teacher to personalize their instructions and provide hands-on assists. Along with classes, he felt it was imperative to develop a home practice that can be done daily. As your home practice is being established, class instruction should continue as new postures are learned that increase strength, flexibility, and endurance. Yoga instruction should not cease with asana, as the path of practice is meant to lead you into other forms of pranayama and eventually the domain of meditation. Over time, a consistent home practice, even if brief, becomes an anchor that informs the whole of your life.

The yogis of old stole away to the forest for good reason. To find time and a quiet place for yoga is very difficult. Today none of us can run away to the woods. In such a situation, how can we manage to progress? An aspiring yogi should work out a convenient schedule that allows for fifteen minutes of daily practice. This much is essential to keep up one's momentum and positive spirit. Morning, noon, and evening are the most favorable times. Starting with fifteen minutes, gradually lengthen the time according to your energy and enthusiasm. Practice steadily and neither be too rapid, nor too slow, in extending the time to one hour. A seasoned student may choose to practice yoga up to a limit of two hours per day. This time may be divided into two or more sessions to suit one's circumstances and convenience.

A PROGRESSIVE PRACTICE

Swami Kripalu taught that in order to stay motivated, your practice needs to deliver results that generate a sense of forward movement. Only then will your enthusiasm for yoga remain vibrant. Here are the ingredients he identified that make a yoga practice *progressive*.

A progressive practice is built upon a solid foundation of theoretical principles and classic techniques that are learned properly from the outset. This ensures initial success and helps avoid disruptions down the road when errors become apparent and fundamentals need to be re-learned. A progressive practice is also aimed at clear goals and performance targets. These goals are set in accord with the known stages of yoga, which over time have proven their ability to produce results. It is only by accomplishing one manageable goal after another that a student gains a growing sense of competence and mastery.

Every yoga practice will include exercises that are done repeatedly because they are consistently beneficial, but a progressive practice is not so repetitive as to become boring. A portion of every session should coax you beyond your comfort zone and into new territory where growth occurs. This results in neurogenesis, the formation of new neural pathways, which is felt as a palpable sense of novelty and aliveness. Progressive practitioners are always experimenting with a few things slightly beyond their current reach in a quest to develop new capacities. This keeps their yoga fresh and avoids any sense of being stuck or stagnant. SK displayed a deep respect for individual differences and taught that yoga can never be a one-size-fits-all endeavor. Every student must feel their way into a practice that meshes with their unique nature and bodily needs. While learning the fundamentals, don't lose sight of the goal to create a personalized practice that works in your life.

Any long-term practice needs to be self-motivated, as external sources of inspiration prove short-lived and eventually peter out. But that doesn't mean your practice should be entirely self-directed. A progressive practice is best overseen by an able teacher who can give ongoing guidance. Ideally, it will also involve peer relationships with a community of like-minded practitioners (sangha) able to offer support and share the transformative journey that consistent yoga practice catalyzes.

SK ON PRACTICE

Achieving radiant health, success in life, and direct spiritual knowledge may sound like an extraordinary task, but these benefits are within reach for anyone willing to engage in regular and deliberate yoga practice.

Practicing yoga aimlessly does not give much pleasure. One performs a routine and receives some benefits but eventually grows disinterested. But a student given proper guidance will feel they are making progress. As a result, they remain interested and practice diligently, which sets them firmly upon the journey of yoga. Such a seeker progresses along the path, gaining the knowledge of yoga through the practice of yoga. This is why it is said in the texts: "Only through the elementary yoga is the advanced yoga generated."

There are many postures, breathing exercises, and meditation methods, but they are not of equal usefulness to everyone. Each student is unique and differs in such things as age, ability, interests, and aspirations. A student must adopt only those techniques that suit his or her nature. To find those techniques, a student should commence a basic practice and listen to the answers that come from within.

The path of yoga reliably leads one to health, good character, and worldly success, but even an individualized practice is best conducted with the guidance of an able teacher. Such a teacher can instruct a student in the correct practice of postures, pranayama, meditation, and other techniques in accord with their capacity. But techniques alone are insufficient for attaining an overall success, which only comes from integrating the principles of yoga into one's personal, family, and work life. A true teacher is one who has attained to this high level through their own practice and gained the ability to model the essence of yoga through the way they live.

TESTED IN LIFE

Yoga practice provides a refuge where you can relax, let your guard down, and take time to self-nurture. Practice can also be a hotbox for growth where you raise energy, explore new realms of self-awareness, and invite new ways of being to emerge. But the yoga you do on your mat and cushion is ultimately a practice—something beneficial done regularly to help you be more connected, present, and effective in your life. That's why SK emphasized that genuine progress in yoga always carries over into daily life:

> *Seekers who practice yoga only in the meditation room are under a great illusion. They must apply its principles in life as well. Yoga techniques are rightly done in the privacy of the meditation room to avoid external disturbances. But exiting the meditation room, one encounters many disturbances, and has to work under great difficulty, and at times persevere in the face of chaos. A true yogi learns in the meditation room and then tests their knowledge in life. This is the path that leads to growth and success.*

BE A DISCERNING STUDENT

Most of SK's Indian students were householders whom he taught to live in accord with the rules of health and principles of dharma. Their primary spiritual practice was mantra yoga linked to their religious faith, as detailed in chapters 18 and 19. Looking back over the centuries-old yoga tradition, the idea of householders doing a daily routine of asana and pranayama appears to be a contemporary phenomenon.

I was already doing yoga postures when I met Swami Kripalu in 1981. Inspired by his example, I commenced a daily three-part practice (asana, pranayama, and meditation) that has deepened over the decades and continues to enrich my life today. Getting on my mat and cushion first thing each morning has served me well, but it's legitimate for a reader to ask, "Is daily practice really necessary? Isn't it sufficient to practice regularly?"

Having only my experience to draw upon, I can't answer this question definitively. I've known some yogis who get up early to practice on workdays, but consider their weekends family time. And others who do a short practice during the week, and dedicate their weekends to going deep. Still others take one day of the week entirely off in the spirit of sabbath. Most just do the best they can, practicing when opportunities present in the midst of their busy lives. Assessing the efficacy of these and other options, it's clear that SK was pointing to something more than a weekly yoga class. Perhaps the answer is that yoga and meditation need to be practiced consistently.

In terms of when to practice, it's worth recounting the experience of the ashram, which strove to make every resident a morning person. After twenty years of shaming natural night-owls for their sporadic 5 a.m. yoga attendance, the administration finally relented and revamped the daily schedule to allow everyone to participate in a late afternoon practice done after work and before dinner.

APPLYING THIS CHAPTER IN PRACTICE

Doing our yoga has become second nature for Danna and me, a part of our morning routine that follows close on the heels of brushing our teeth. If that kind of consistency sounds daunting, most psychologists agree that it is not as hard as we think to form new and healthier habits. Although exactly how long that takes is debatable. Some cite the 21/90 Rule, which says it takes twenty-one days to form a habit and ninety days to transform that habit into a permanent lifestyle change. Others refer to research that suggests the entire process takes six-months or more. Regardless of who's right, it's clear the power of automaticity eventually begins to work for you. This is important, as good health habits including what medical doctors call "exercise adherence" is a vital component of lasting wellness.

While getting into a groove is a good first step, that does not mean your work to sustain a vital yoga practice is done. In all forms of repetitive behavior, a groove eventually becomes a rut. That just means it's time to shake things up. Perhaps you've been enjoying a particular routine of postures, pranayama, and meditation. If that starts feeling stale, try switching the order. Begin with pranayama, then move into postures. Or meditate first thing, before your mind gets activated, and continue from there. A willingness to shift gears and "do different" is an essential part of keeping your practice alive and engaging.

A dedicated yogi moving through the stages of yoga should expect their practice to exhibit a mix of steadiness and dynamism. For example, practice is likely to start out as posture-based with pranayama playing a supportive role. At some point, pranayama may step into the limelight, with asana practice playing a still-important but auxiliary role. Later on, meditation is likely to be front and center, with breath and movement practices continued to nurture bodily health and prepare the mind to move through the stages of dharana, dhyana, and samadhi.

In an evolving practice, new tools and techniques appear as needed to spark growth in a particular area. Some of this novelty may be self-generated, arising intuitively from inner knowing. Others tools may come from outside as different teachers and teachings draw your interest. Once that growth has happened, it is fine to let these subsidiary practices fall away. It is counterproductive to keep repeating techniques that for a time generated forward movement growth, but after completing their useful life stop working.

Early in his treatise, sage Patanjali says the first five limbs of yoga (yama, niyama, asana, pranayama, and pratyahara) are supports for the last three limbs – dharana, dhyana, and samadhi. Later in his treatise, dharana and dhyana are said to be supports for samadhi, as only through samadhi does the mind dissolve into the atman or self. This is not an inconsistency. In the same way that an aspirant's mind will pass through many states on the path to attaining spiritual knowledge, the yogic techniques they adopt as means to progress will similarly change. The primary practices (asana, pranayama, meditation) are like the commanders of an army, as their task is to purify and enliven the entire system so energy can build and move upwards. To accomplish this purpose, they are done continuously but with greater and greater subtlety.

Other kriyas (actions taken in practice) are like foot soldiers. They appear to help win a specific battle and disappear forever. Lower forms of practice are replaced by higher forms of practice – an aspirant must understand this principle to enter the deeper spheres of yoga.

Looking back, I certainly could have been more purposeful in my practice. It's embarrassing how long it took me to figure out what the techniques I was doing every morning were really meant to accomplish. If an opportunity had presented to work closely with a teacher like Swami Kripalu, it is possible I would have progressed light years faster, but that's just speculation. The truth is a path of steady practice and gradual self-development has been good for me. Forty years into it and now in my mid-sixties, yoga is still bringing forth new and surprising capacities in me. SK might have said, "Of course, that reflects the science of yoga." As for me, I find it miraculous.

We believe we know what potentials are hidden within us, but that is a faulty notion. A person may be aware that he is a fast runner, but then discover he can go faster when he runs not alone but with others. This may lead him to test himself in competition and determine his utmost speed limit, but again this is not true. Returning home from a scary movie on a dark night, he imagines some foe is coming to kill him and runs faster than ever before. Great people who know yoga say that there are numberless secrets and countless mysteries hidden in your body and mind that can be discovered through practice. Where do these hidden potentials come from? They all come from your root life energy and spiritual source. Yoga teaches you how to activate that energy and bring forth that source.

CHAPTER 14
HEALTHY LIVING

Through the regular practice of yoga, bit by bit, the body and mind are rearranged and a change in your basic nature occurs that makes you want to live a healthy and spiritually-elevating life.

In the fall of 1982, all the ashram residents piled into a caravan of cars and trucks bound for the Berkshire Hills of western Massachusetts. The burgeoning community was moving to a more-spacious facility, a former Jesuit novitiate that had been vacant for decades. Its towering brick edifice was built on a hillside overlooking a picturesque lake. After several months of dawn-to-dark work, the reconstituted ashram opened its doors as the Kripalu Center for Yoga & Health. I was a third-year law student and money was tight, but Danna and I managed to scrape together the registration fees for one of its initial program offerings, a weekend retreat entitled "Journey to Holistic Health."

On opening night, I learned that the Pennsylvania ashram had been a hub in the grassroots holistic health movement that swept the country in the 1970s. At the heart of the movement was a simple idea. Health is more than the absence of disease; it's a positive state of wellness that naturally arises when body, mind, and spirit are in harmony. Combating illness with drugs and surgery makes little sense when often it can be prevented by common-sense measures like diet, exercise, positive thinking, and stress management. Instead of bowing to experts from the medical establishment, holistic health encourages individuals to take responsibility for their own well-being. As the program unfolded, I began to see how the ashram faculty was grafting a new branch of yoga onto the tree of holistic health. One handout made this exceedingly clear:

True health is more than eating right, quitting smoking, or jogging every day. It's a state of radiant well-being. Holistic health is an effort to experience what the ancient Greeks had in mind when they coined the word "holos," an experience of a wholeness that borders on holiness, with body, mind and spirit in a triune affirmation of our fullest potential. This kind of health does not end with having a finely tuned body or even a calm and perceptive mind. It seeks to merge all aspects of ourselves in the high levels of energetic aliveness, inner peace, joy, and spiritual illumination for which we were born. As whole and integrated beings, we have the potential to reach an apex that transcends normalcy. Health is not truly holistic unless and until it encompasses this ascent towards the realm that yoga calls Self-realization.

Once alerted to these ideas linking health and yoga, I began to find their seeds scattered throughout SK's teachings:

Illness seldom enters our life without an invitation. The invitation usually comes through some form of improper living. The first remedy for any problem is healthy lifestyle with care taken to address symptoms through wholesome diet, regular exercise, and restful sleep. Postures, pranayama, and yogic relaxation can be very helpful, as their practice revitalizes the nerves, organs and glands. Medicines can also be useful, especially to remedy serious conditions, but they should be used only when natural measures fail to eradicate the root cause of disease. When doctors teach the science of healthy living, our hospitals will turn into true temples of health.

It's been forty years since that pioneering program. The upstart ideas central to holistic health are now mainstream and embraced by established professional fields including complementary and alternative medicine, functional medicine, and positive psychology. Fueled by popular interest, the ingredients of a healthy lifestyle have been rigorously researched, and the findings hotly debated. Current studies often point out the role played by genetic diversity in everyday matters including the topics featured in this chapter: diet, exercise, and sleep. While doing my best to keep up with the rapidly evolving research, I continue to find the age-old outlook of the yoga tradition helpful, as it presents the building blocks of health in a way that enables practitioners to assemble them into a synergistic whole greater than any of its parts.

SK ON HEALTHY LIFESTYLE

We all must travel the long distance of a lifetime in this body. If we do not care for it, how can we reach our goal? Without a body, we would not be able to perform a single action. With a body that is fit, we can perform many actions effectively. Until the body is healthy, other approaches to growth cannot help us much because the cause of an unruly mind is often an ailing body. This is why the yogis teach that cultivating bodily health is the best means of attaining spirituality. Truly, it can be said that the end of disease is the first step in yoga.

All the organs and glands are strengthened by the practice of proper diet, regular exercise, good sleep, and yoga. If their function is weak, one's health suffers. If their function is adequate, one enjoys the disease-free state. If their function is strong, one reaches maximum development. We don't suspect that a superior person can emerge from an ailing person through these simple practices. We don't believe that we can achieve success in our worldly and spiritual endeavors through right living. This is why it's important to have faith in the yogic approach and never abandon these practices.

I was afraid of disease; now disease is afraid of me. Health had forsaken me in anger; now it is pleased and remains always with me. I was ignorant and blinded by the dark shadow of worry, but the fountain of knowledge has burst forth, and now the bright light of intuition is illuminating the path of my life. This is not imaginative fantasy. It is the description of a stage of yoga born from a regular practice that will unfailingly bless you with a sense of good health, emotional buoyancy, mental fearlessness, and enthusiasm for life.

A recent *Time* magazine cover proclaimed that it contained "the secrets of happiness experts." Several articles were grouped in a section called "The Happiness Revival Guide" which explained how our brains are wired to be good at many things, but making us happy isn't one of them. For example, after a long day, your brain might recommend a pint of ice cream and a night of binge watching, when you would be much better served by resisting the urge to zone out and going to bed early.

This kind of mismatch between what we think will make us happy and what truly works is a big contributor to what the experts point to as our rampant unhappiness. People across the board believe that happiness will come with good grades, a high-paying job, and ascending to higher social status. But the research tells a different story. What actually makes people happy are activities that promote physical health and mental well-being. Bodily, this involves getting adequate sleep, regular exercise, and good nutrition. The mental factors cited include nurturing family and community relationships, cultivating an attitude of gratitude, finding ways to foster mindfulness such as walks in nature and meditation, and engaging in socially-beneficial pursuits that instill everyday life with meaning and purpose.

I finished those articles grateful for the teachings I'd been steering my life by for decades, as SK's path of yoga contain all the elements featured by their happiness experts and more.

In ancient India, the yogis gave the topic of diet deep consideration and regarded it as tremendously important because they knew a person's physical and mental energy must be protected by right eating. Proper diet was thus considered foundational to yoga. Any approach to healing, growth, and awakening that is unconcerned with diet is not a true science and will not survive for long.

EATING WELL

Learning to eat well is probably the single most powerful thing you can do to improve your quality of life. While an ardent advocate for healthy eating, SK refrained from recommending any particular diet. He considered food choice a highly personal matter, a riddle every person must solve by experimentation. Instead of prescribing what to eat, he taught a step-by-step method of learning how to eat.

It's easy to fall into a pattern of habitual, unconscious, and often anxious eating. The first step in eating well is breaking out of this rut by remaining self-aware and present in your body during the act of eating. Conscious eating is more pleasurable than wolfing your food, as it requires you to slow down, chew each bite, and pay attention to all the sights, smells, and tastes. Creating the conditions to relax at mealtimes is key, as lingering stress inhibits the digestive process.

> *Eating food that you like is one of the pleasures of life, and all of us can learn to eat in a way that protects our health. Choose foods that are good for your body and eat them on a regular schedule. Chew your food well, mixing it thoroughly with saliva. Do not fill the stomach completely. Leave a little extra space to support good digestion. Between meals, try not to eat unless you are truly hungry. Allow your stomach to be empty for a while so the digestive process can complete. Stay conscious when you sit down at the table and stop eating when you've satisfied your hunger. While eating too much brings yawns and makes the mind cranky, eating moderately preserves your alertness and bestows an after-meal joy.*

Once grounded in the practice of conscious eating, you can take a second step by starting to eat with what SK calls *discrimination*. Gradually wean yourself away from less-than-healthy foods by replacing them with more wholesome options. Instead of denying yourself, delight in the process of discerning what foods are truly good for you. Notice what you actually enjoy eating, and also how you feel and perform afterwards. Don't lose sight of the fact that a healthy diet is more than a matter of nutritional content and calories. SK recognized that our emotional needs and preferences play a vital role in satiation and satisfaction. When you've learned what foods really work, eat them with gratitude. And stay awake to the process, as your needs are always changing.

> *An aspiring yogi abandons indiscriminate eating and adopts a wholesome diet. In this practice, one eats to nourish the entire being rather than satisfy only the taste buds. A wholesome diet consists of foods and dishes that are both healthy and tasty. It has a good texture, being neither too dry nor too wet, and is thus easy to digest. It avoids extreme foods that irritate the stomach or otherwise upset the digestive process. A wholesome diet must also take into*

consideration one's emotions, as the body and mind are intricately related, so the foods you eat should be pleasing to the heart. This type of diet, when eaten with gratitude and love for life, will generate a balance of good health, vigor, and happiness.

EXERCISE

Swami Kripalu echoes the Greek sage Hippocrates, who is considered the father of western medicine and said, "Eating alone will not keep a man well. He must also take exercise." Anyone intent on improving their diet soon discovers the need to balance food consumption with physical activity. If we broaden our definition of eating well to include efficient digestion and elimination, the role of exercise as an essential element in the equation of good health becomes apparent.

SK ON THE RELATIONSHIP OF DIET AND EXERCISE

I will now explain the complementary relationship between exercise, food, and health. If we don't get enough exercise, our food does not digest completely. Waste products are not excreted fully and go on collecting, toxifying the body and causing ill health. Thus, exercise is just as necessary for health as food and water. Anyone who grasps this physiological fact will find ways to make it part of their daily routine. If you wish to speak the language of health, you must know that food is the noun and exercise is the verb.

Exercise creates a natural appetite. When a person eats with real appetite, even a dry crust of bread tastes delicious. On the other hand, when a sedentary person eats from habit, even the richest foods seem tasteless. Anyone eating wholesome foods who chews thoroughly and exercises regularly soon discovers that these three practices not only uproot the tree of disease but saturate life with happiness and joy.

On days we exercise little, our appetite is naturally reduced. On days we exercise a lot, our appetite is increased. In this way, each meal tests our powers of discrimination, and we must gauge how much we need to eat by how much we have exerted ourselves that day. When we eat and exercise in proportion, our food digests properly. We sleep deeply and do not have disturbing dreams. When awake we remain alert and in a pleasant mood. If these conditions are created, progress in yoga comes easily.

Long before SK began practicing yoga postures, he walked several miles a day and did pushups and other calisthenics to keep fit. While hatha yoga is sometimes touted as "the most perfect form of exercise," he saw value in aerobic conditioning, strength training, and many other types of physical culture. The following excerpt culls his guidance into a compact teaching explaining why *exercise is rightly considered part of yoga*.

> *Any fitness seeker wanting to enjoy the pleasures of good health is actually a beginning yogi. The moment we hear the word "exercise" we think of bodily exertion because it's commonly associated with vigorous activities that work the muscles. But exercise is best defined as intentional activity that increases the rate of respiration. Any form of movement performed with full awareness will bring favorable results. This includes walking, running, swimming, calisthenics, and weight lifting. Sports require a special mental focus, which stimulates brain centers. Active games add the element of fun and laughter, which causes us to momentarily forget our problems and fosters healing. Dance brings heartfelt joy, and the rhythmic breathing of singing bestows bliss. The aftereffects of activities like these can influence a person for days at a time.*
>
> *While different types of exercise produce different results, all have in common the purpose of preventing disease and preserving health. Instead of taking medicine right away to remedy our discomforts, it is better to eat right and exercise. Most of us know this is the best path. But in many forms of exercise there is a sense of dryness and boredom. Even a person who loves to exercise will lapse into periods of doing it unconsciously. It is hard to find much joy in mindless repetition and the benefit of exercises done mechanically also decreases. Finding ways to counteract this tendency is important, which is why I believe that every yoga ashram should have a gymnasium and playground. It's important for farmers and those doing physical labor all day long to know that other forms of bodily*

exercise are not necessary for them. Manual workers need to give rest to the body. It is those laboring with their brains who require physical exercise to give rest to the mind.

It is narrow-minded to think that yoga lives only in temples and prayer halls. Good health is a need of everyone, and yoga practice must begin as physical exercise to serve a broad range of people. Yoga must put on the dress of exercise; then only will the world become healthy, happy, and spiritually inclined. Find exercises that suit your body and temperament and practice them daily.

SK advised beginning students to establish themselves in a pattern of wholesome eating and some appealing form of regular exercise. Once this foundation was laid, the systematic practice of yoga could carry them beyond their particular predilections and into entirely new territory.

Yoga is a comprehensive system that develops the body and mind in a balanced fashion. Lovers of physical exercise develop their muscles until they are fit and firm, but their exclusive focus on the body can prevent them from developing their minds. Intellectuals call these people "jocks." Lovers of mental acumen develop their brainpower, but their exclusive focus on the mind can prevent them from developing physical strength. Jocks call these people "eggheads." On the path of yoga, one first adopts the practice of physical exercise to establish bodily fitness. Next one learns yogic breathing and uses various postures to harmonize the respiratory, nervous, and circulatory systems, which increases overall vitality. Then one engages the subtle exercises of concentration and meditation to develop the powers of the mind. Yoga's uniqueness is that it ultimately carries one beyond body and mind to Atman, the singlular source of body and mind that energizes every thought and action.

REVITALIZING SLEEP

Accustomed as many of us are to burning the candle at both ends, it can be challenging to get enough rest. As science studies sleep, a growing body of research is making it clear that adequate and deep sleep is a pillar of health on par with diet and exercise. Sleep has been shown to boost mood, improve memory, aid learning, ease stress, curb inflammation, sharpen attention, spur creativity, enhance effectiveness, increase stamina, reduce daytime fatigue, and help avoid accidents. Sleep also helps us maintain healthy body weight by moderating appetite and easing hunger cravings. In all these and other ways, good sleep helps us live better and longer.

When sleep is deficient, studies reveal that our health is at risk. A connection has been established between inadequate sleep and a host of conditions including adult-onset diabetes; cardiovascular problems including high blood pressure, high cholesterol, and heart attacks; strokes; impaired immune response; obesity; depression and mood disorders; alcoholism; and a reduced ability to concentrate that results in poor cognitive function. The degree of impairment exhibited by drivers who have not slept well is causing safety experts to point out sleep deficits as a public health hazard equal to drunk driving.

How can a good night's sleep do so many things? Long before any of this research could be conducted, the yogis observed that while sleeping the body and brain are freed from other responsibilities to focus their full energies on the tasks associated with healing and health maintenance.

> *During the day, our minds are active in controlling the body's voluntary systems to accomplish our work in the world. Hard work is taxing to the body, and this situation is compounded if the mind is worried about the success or failure of its plans, which keeps the nervous system tense. With our energy directed externally, we cannot attend very well to the needs of our internal environment. At night when the mind falls asleep, our bodily energy is free to do its inner work. During sleep, the brain and all the bodily organs and glands are purified of wastes. Depleted cells are replenished, damaged cells are replaced, and many other essential tasks are performed. All these tasks are best done without any interference of mind, which is why sound sleep is so necessary. Lacking this rest, people are prone to sickness and suffer mental and emotional problems. Sleep is a gift of nature and the finest medicine to maintain good health. When nature is reminding you of the need for sleep by making your head*

nod and mouth yawn, give heed to its call and go to bed grateful for its desire to protect your health.

One of the most interesting discoveries of the past decade is that the brain has a waste management system that removes metabolic wastes from the cerebral tissues during deep dreamless or non-REM (rapid eye movement) sleep. There is some evidence suggesting that chronic deep-sleep deprivation hinders the function of this glymphatic system and might play a role in brain disorders including Alzheimer's disease and dementia. The dreaming that occurs in REM sleep is known to play an important neurological role in learning and memory consolidation, the process whereby new memories are transferred into long-term storage.

Psychologist Ernest Rossi takes this a step further by noting that the human psyche is a dynamic system. It's commonplace for people to have one part of their personality actively in conflict with another, which is known to undermine happiness and drive harmful behavior. Rossi believes that one function of dreaming is to help integrate these separate psychological structures into a more harmonious and comprehensive personality. According to Rossi, sleep and dreaming are the natural means through which ongoing personality development takes place.

SK ON THE GODDESS OF SLEEP

After the day's toil, we lay our body down and are visited by the merciful goddess of sleep. This goddess truly has a mother's love. She takes us in her lap and lovingly strokes our head to break our contact with the external world and free us from pain. As we dream, she plays us sweet and soothing melodies. When our whole body has come to rest in the depths of dreamless sleep, she accomplishes many healing tasks. She also renews our mind. If we fall asleep depressed or disappointed, she inspires us. If we are troubled by a problem, she gives us glimpses of the knowledge that will satisfy our need for an answer. And just as a mother educates her child, so also mother sleep makes us a spiritual seeker by instilling in us a complete faith that going within is the way to real happiness, peace, and liberation. Truly this goddess of sleep is the servant of everyone.

Yoga says that there are three states of mind we all know: the waking state, the dream state, and the state of dreamless sleep.

Beyond these three is what yoga calls the fourth (turiya), also known as samadhi. The true rest bestowed by a thought-free mind can only be found in deep dreamless sleep or samadhi. Without sleep, the world would be full of mental patients and it would be impossible to enjoy a long and healthy life. Without samadhi, it would be impossible to reach the atman (soul). Indeed, the depths of yogic meditation can be understood as a process of penetrating the sleep states with awareness.

A DAILY ROUTINE

Swami Kripalu's teachings on lifestyle are grounded in Ayurveda, India's indigenous system of medicine. Ayurveda means "science of living" and it places great emphasis on the role of establishing a daily routine (*dinacharya*) to promote health. Ideally, the day begins with a natural wake-up time that leads directly into morning hygiene. That is followed by self-care practices like yoga, meditation, and time outside in nature. Mindful meals and a degree of consistency in work hours and exercise is seen as necessary to regularize the processes of digestion, absorption, assimilation, and elimination. The day ends with a consistent bed time that ensures adequate sleep. Along with maintaining internal balance, a daily routine was believed to keep one's biological clock synchronized with the nature's circadian rhythms. Over time the practice of dinacharya was credited with ordering one's life in a way that generated a sense of agency, purpose, self-esteem and spiritual attunement accompanied by feelings of inner peace and outer happiness.

SK ON DAILY ROUTINE

Whatever I wish to practice, I find a way to fit into my daily schedule. One day I was sitting on my porch swing after lunch when it dawned on me that Ayurveda advises a person to walk at least one hundred steps after eating. This was simple enough for me to do, and I knew it would be good for me. I immediately got up and walked around my dwelling place seven times. For years, I've continued this practice and enjoyed its many benefits. If you want to prosper materially and spiritually, follow a regular schedule that helps you not only remain healthy but fulfill your daily obligations with a tranquil mind. This schedule should include bathing daily, as the skin has millions of pores that need to be kept open to perspire freely. Through perspiration one eliminates unnecessary salts and oils. Dust particles come into contact with this perspiration and stick to the body. If a person does not bathe regularly, the skin accumulates layers of dirt that close the pores and make one vulnerable to ill health. Daily bathing is not a religious ritual for yogis; it has a practical purpose.

MAKE TIME TO PLAY

One element highlighted in that initial holistic health program surprised me. An entire afternoon session was dedicated to play and humor. At the time, I was a serious spiritual seeker. All these years later, I still struggle with that malady. A program handout captioned "The Way of Play" spoke directly to this:

> No one has to teach children how to play or laugh or take time to have some fun. They come into this world experiencing everything anew and delighted by the simplest things. In growing up, most of us have lost these qualities. We've become too busy to play. Play and humor are essential to holistic health, as it's precisely when we get too serious about life that we experience the negative effects of stress. All we need do is consciously rediscover the child within us. Children can make fun out of almost anything. A few pebbles become a castle, a little breeze and a kite have endless possibilities. We've got to remember how to let go of our day-to-day cares and play again. At first, you'll have to schedule it into your grown-up life. Maybe it's as simple as a game of softball or volleyball. Start today and you'll soon find your pressures and struggles consumed by the innocent joy of laughter and fun. Seeing how serious you've become you'll have a good belly laugh at yourself and in the process rekindle the attitude that makes everything a great undiscovered mystery.

Returning home, I was even more surprised to find this advice mirrored in the teachings of SK. Rather than brush it aside as workshop fluff, I had to take notice:

Before I became a swami, I used to go out and play with the village children whenever my mind was disturbed. By becoming one of them, and giving them laughter, I would laugh too. The result was that I regained my peace and happiness. This is how I learned the beautiful role of play in life. Now I am a swami, but I haven't stopped playing tricks and creating innocent mischief. If you want to free your mind from all worries, learn to play. Yoga eventually teaches all of us that seriousness is a high crime in the court of God.

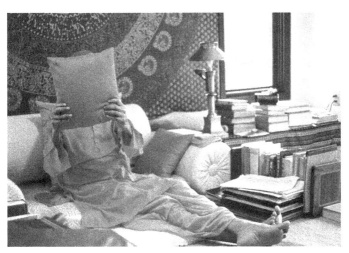

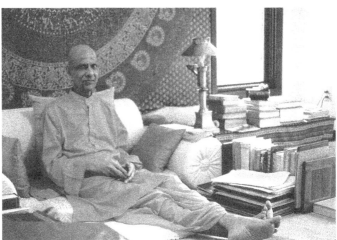

When an ashram photographer was dispatched to take some shots of Swami Kripalu relaxing in his residence, his first response was mischievous. After they shared a good laugh, he relented to having his picture taken.

THE BUILDING BLOCKS OF HEALTH

Long before the advent of the holistic health movement in America, SK was teaching his students the building blocks of health as presented in this chapter, which he collectively called a *yogic lifestyle*. Along with teaching these practices, he modeled their application in life and was always on the lookout for ways to optimize his daily routine:

> *I learned a trick of how to remain fresh and productive from the lower caste women of India, who often smoke. There are good reasons for this habit. They have to work very hard doing the same thing all day long. Suffering this drudgery, they get tired and have no other justification to sit down and take rest other than smoking. This reason is accepted by their employers and gives them a few precious moments of relaxation. Seeing that I also need to rest, but knowing that creating an addiction is not an answer, I pondered what to do and eventually found a solution. If I am studying yoga and get tired, I shift to music. When I become bored with that, I go into meditation. Whenever one of my likings temporarily becomes a disliking, I take to another liking to remove my fatigue and mental restlessness. This is my method of refreshment and it continually renews my enthusiasm.*

A year after our first holistic health retreat, Danna and I spent a summer at Kripalu Center as volunteers in "Spiritual Lifestyle Training," a three-month program designed to provide an in-depth experience of yogic living. That experience eventually led us to join the residential staff, which worked hard in the spirit of karma yoga (the yoga of skillful action), but also enjoyed a smorgasbord of vegetarian foods, early morning and afternoon yoga classes, a fully-equipped fitness facility, and a basement full of bicycles. Each day at lunchtime, the offices emptied and staff members headed out to walk, jog, run, dance, in-line skate, swim in the lake, or take part in a pickup soccer or volleyball game. There was a fall triathlon, which many residents trained for all year, as well an annual work retreat that ended with "fun day," a twenty-four-hour extravaganza of pranks, skits, musical performances, and ice cream sundaes.

After becoming residents, Danna was immediately assigned to the programs department, where she supported a three-week retreat that was the premier offering in Kripalu Center's guest curriculum. The Health for Life program taught the basics of healthy living to groups of twenty participants who worked directly with a team of vegetarian chefs, medical doctors, yoga instructors, and experts in lifestyle change. All of this was a reflection of SK's positive spirit, which saw progress on the path of yoga as a natural outgrowth of healthy living.

A yogic lifestyle has the power to eradicate all kinds of disease, but it still takes discipline to acquire the clarity, strength, and energy of good health. Once your direction has been set, concern yourself solely with your day-to-day activities. Your only thought should be, "How much can I progress today?" Thinking this way, your enthusiasm will steadily increase. A wall is built stone by stone, and a lake can be filled drop by drop. In the same way, you can best make your journey to health by focusing on your immediate progress.

CHAPTER 15
LOVE IN THE FAMILY

If you don't want to practice yoga—then don't! But if you wish to live happily in this world, you will have to learn how to love those closest to you. There is nothing more important that I could ever tell you.

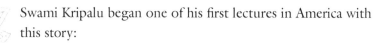

Swami Kripalu began one of his first lectures in America with this story:

> In the India in which I grew up, it was not uncommon for a holy man to arrive in a town or city and loudly announce, "I have a secret! One thing I have learned from my life, that I want to tell before I die, and I'll take 10,000 rupees for it." Today it is difficult for us to understand how the experiential knowledge gained by a holy man like this could be so valuable, but back then there would be people willing to buy it. After taking the 10,000 rupees, the holy man would give a teaching that he had ardently practiced to attain success, and he would say it very directly in a single sentence. You might be surprised that a holy man would do this, and feel that he was just robbing his customer, but this is not the case. It was known that any purchaser who took such a teaching to heart would be well satisfied. Were I that holy man, and you the customer, I would tell you, "Love your family, and grow from there." That single sentence is more valuable than 10,000 rupees, and it is my gift to you.

SK was a product of village India, where the extended family was the dominant social and economic structure. Looking through this lens, he saw the family unit as the critical link in a chain that bound the well-being of individuals to the welfare of society. If a family is healthy and prosperous, it produces happy children. As young men and women, they are apt to grow into hard-working citizens willing to contribute to the collective good and continue the virtuous cycle as caring parents. In his mind, there was no getting around the fact that the only way to populate society with able adults is to fortify the family. He believed this simple logic governed the success of communities, nations, and civilization itself.

Unfortunately, its converse was equally true. If the chain is broken at the link of family, everyone suffers:

When a person is born into a troubled family, his thirsty heart cannot drink in love and negative traits are tattooed all over his mind. Unable to trust his loved ones, he finds it difficult to trust anyone else, and everyone's troubles multiply from there. Our homes are not just houses; they are the schoolrooms of culture. While the word culture is on the lips of many politically-minded people these days, few of them know how to establish it in their own lives. Every culture has its roots in families and their method of living. For a society to truly progress, it must uplift the family. This is why love in the family is my most favorite principle.

Along with the good feelings that accompany it, love was a moral imperative to Swami Kripalu, a duty arising from the fact of our interrelatedness. He felt this obligation is self-evident and requires no explanation because it already lives deep in every person's heart. All that is needed is a little encouragement to bring it forth. The love of which he spoke was not the romantic variety so front and center today. It is a genuine warmth and caring for the welfare of others. An active effort is required to become a loving person, a lifelong learning process that starts with the members of our immediate family and steadily expands outward to embrace all of humanity.

SK didn't back away from the fact that authentic love requires a lot from us. First, we must overcome the inertia of our self-interest by paying attention to the wants and needs of others. Then we have to hone our ability to listen, relate positively, and communicate with sensitivity and affection. Even while pursuing our own ends, we must take the preferences of others into consideration. Finally, we have to take action, as love remains mere sentimentality until it's expressed in tangible ways that serve the interests of our loved ones.

To maintain peace in the home, we must take up the practice of speaking lovingly. Sweet speech invites togetherness, where harsh speech causes others to run away from us. Everyone knows this, but to truly speak lovingly we must also learn to digest responses to our words that are difficult for us to hear. These two practices go together; we cannot do one without the other. Otherwise, our sweet speech will immediately leave us when a sibling, spouse, or child points out a blind spot or shortcoming. It is important to remember that our inadequacies are apparent to the people that surround us. When a loving family member reveals an area of weakness, we must learn to listen and trust that they are giving us needed guidance.

The ability of people to remain unaware of their real motives and mistaken about the likability of their personality has long been known. The ancient Greeks described humanity as blinded by hubris. Poets and playwrights have observed that people see themselves through rose-colored spectacles. Religious thinkers have cautioned us not to adopt a holier than thou attitude in which we are quick to criticize others but avoid looking at our own warts and blemishes. Christ distilled this teaching into a powerful soundbite: "Why do you point out the speck in your brother's eye but fail to see the log in your own eye?" (Matthew 7:3)

More recently, social psychologists have shown that we mentally go to great lengths to view the world in a way that maintains our self-esteem and sense of moral superiority. It appears the strength of our need to feel good about ourselves is sufficient to render us unable to see our deficits. This is why Swami Kripalu valued the mirroring provided by others, which offers us a perspective that is not obscured by our defensive rationalizations and justifications. Psychologists agree with the wisdom of this approach, saying that it is often better to deduce our real motivations by looking at our behavior and how others react to us. Although SK felt this was a serious lesson for a truth seeker to learn, he made his point by telling two humorous stories.

Dwelling on the faults of others prevents you from seeing your own shortcomings. This is a real block to progress. Once it so happened that a colander and a needle got together. The colander's gaze fell on the needle's eye and she said out loud, "Oh, the needle has a hole!" Then the colander looked down to find innumerable holes in herself and was ashamed.

In the East, a camel is described as the animal with eighteen curves. Once one of these camels saw a dog and thought to himself, "Such a curved tail!" So the camel went close and said, "Oh, poor dog, you have such a curvy body." The dog asked, "What part of me is curved?" The camel said, "Ah, you don't even know that? Your tail is curved." The dog looked carefully at every one of the camel's curves. His eyes went up eighteen times, and his eyes went down eighteen times, but he said nothing in response.

The moral of these stories is one and the same. Look only for the good qualities in others and be quick to see your own faults. That way your progress on the spiritual path will be swift and sure.

At the outset of my studies, I was as clueless as the proverbial colander and camel. How did SK's teachings on love in the family related to yoga? The two topics seemed worlds apart. Fortunately, I didn't let that stop me from taking his guidance to heart. Part of my willingness to put these ideas into practice was my painful starting place. Once off to college, my relationship with my parents grew distant and strained. Our differences began over superficial things. They did not like my long hair, vegetarian diet, and penchant for hitchhiking. But as I began to make decisions that would determine the course of my life, the conflict grew more substantive. They questioned my choices, calling them starry-eyed and impractical.

I responded defiantly, proclaiming my alternative values like a broken record. They got fed up with what sounded like an attempt to win them over to my way of thinking. I felt hurt by their disappointment, which they voiced in an attempt to get me back on a mainstream track. As I went my own way, things spiraled downward. My parents weren't impressed by the starting salary of the legal services job I took after law school. Closer to the bone, they attacked my choice of a mate, something that drove a wedge between them and me.

In the course of daily life together, differences in opinion and disputes will arise between family members. Patience, respect, and tolerance should be used to remove the source of conflict and prevent it from escalating. Remember in these situations that our speech can be like poison or nectar. Where bodily hurts heal quickly, the wounds inflicted by poisonous words do not heal for a very long time. This is why we must be vigilant to not allow the friction of superficial disagreements to cause deeper divisions in the hearts of our family members.

A few years into our marriage, things got even worse when Danna and I moved into Kripalu Center, which my parents labeled a cult. This was my sorry state of affairs when I began studying SK's teachings on love in the family. My emotional estrangement from my parents was close to complete at this point. I went through the motions of keeping in touch but had abandoned any hope of a real relationship. But as I took these teachings to heart and made an effort to lower my defenses, my parents reciprocated. I could tell that they didn't want to lose me entirely. Even in this difficult setting, we began to find the common ground upon which our former closeness could renew itself. When Danna and I moved out of the ashram, they lent us money to buy a house, which we paid back with regular letters home and checks that included a fair rate of interest.

It took years, but over time the situation totally changed. Danna and I did little things to help out after my mother suffered a stroke. That continued through her two decades of limited mobility, increasing deafness, and worsening dementia. My father became her round-the-clock caregiver, and our role became one of supporting him and cheering her up with regular visits. By the time my mother died in 2014, the four of us had not only healed our rifts but grown dear to one another. Ten years later, my father is ninety-nine and still living independently. Our father-son relationship has never been stronger, and Danna is like a daughter to him.

Looking back, I know that my side of this miracle has its roots in teachings like the following:

The first requisite in spiritual life is that peace reign in your household. If there is no peace at home, your mind will always be disturbed. If your household is peaceful, your buoyancy and mental equilibrium will be preserved, and you can face and overcome any disturbances that crop up. To establish peace, you will have to win the hearts of every individual—no matter how big or small—as any peace established by force is but a reign of terror. Only after tuning an instrument can we sing with it. Only after establishing harmony in your family is the chanting of the spiritual life possible.

The root cause of family conflict is fault finding. Instead of ruminating on negativity, cultivate the habit of appreciating the other. Where blame finds fault, love sees virtue. Virtue-finders inspire loved ones by example, showing goodwill and affection. Where a coercive person compulsively harasses, the loving personality uplifts and does not seek to dominate. If conflict increases daily through fault finding, the vine of love withers and eventually disappears. If love increases daily through positive appreciation, its flowers bloom and spread its sweet fragrance everywhere. When affection pervades a family, how happy that family is!

For now, let us put aside any thoughts of loving the whole world. Let's focus our efforts on loving the members of our own family. After learning to love our family, it will become simple for us to love others, as a heart engrossed in familial love will spontaneously love the world.

Alongside family interactions, village life in India took place within a rich web of community relationships. SK taught that people who learned to love their family would grow to radiate respect and caring to everyone with whom they interacted. As my family woes lessened, I actively wanted to be that kind of person, a helper and well-wisher of all. Once I saw that there was a path to becoming a more loving person, I did my best to walk it and not just at home. As SK taught:

Peace is equally necessary in your field of work outside the house. You must make all your pastimes cordial by your positive personality, polite speech, straightforwardness, tolerance for differences in thinking and conduct, and the habit of giving importance to others. These qualities are magnetic and will attract others toward you. If you can get your colleagues in a cooperative mood, your work will become easy, but only genuine love can win the hearts of others. Love is not a business deal. It seeks no profit or reward and serves without coercion. Yet it can truly be said that if you want to meet with true success, learn to love.

Swami Kripalu greeting children before a public lecture in America. Much of the charitable work he spearheaded in India provided basic health care and vocational education to children from less-advantaged families.

We need this approach now more than ever before, when today's public health advocates have declared social isolation the epidemic of our time. Over forty-percent of Americans report feeling lonely, which research correlates with a higher risk of major illness including heart disease, stroke, depression, anxiety, dementia, and premature death from all causes. The net effect is a reduction of lifespan on par with smoking and obesity. And the negative consequences of loneliness extend beyond the doctor's office. At work and school, it lowers task performance, limits creativity, impairs reasoning, inhibits decision making, and reduces executive function.

Research efforts are underway to identify the causal connection between loneliness and all these maladies. Psychologists theorize that humans evolved as highly social creatures living in tight-knit tribes and family units. Banding together was essential to survival, making us hard wired to be socially bonded. Perhaps as a result, the body registers feelings of loneliness as a threat, which raises our level of cortisol and other stress chemicals. This disturbs sleep, inhibits brain function, and suppresses the immune response, leaving us prone to colds, infections, and other minor ailments. If the stress of loneliness is prolonged through significant periods of social isolation, it triggers a cascade of negative physiological and psychological effects that lowers our quality of life and shaves an estimated eight years off life expectancy. More studies are needed on the health value of networking technologies, but at this point it does not appear that social media offers a remedy. Electronic interaction alone is insufficient to relieve our feeling of isolation. Seeing people daily, nurturing friendships, having an emotional confidant and playing that role for others, intimacies like these appear essential to our well-being. The truth of all this was painfully confirmed by the COVID-19 pandemic.

It's hard to know how SK would have responded to the modern family, which was only beginning to take shape during his lifetime. He was a proponent of the traditional family, which in India operated with a rigid set of cultural norms established to preserve its homogeneity and undergird a hierarchically-structured society. Today's families are increasingly diverse. With a frequency hard to imagine a generation ago, people of different races, social classes, religious faiths, and ethnic backgrounds intermarry. In recent decades, it's become commonplace for men to marry other men, and women other women. Right now, the whole notion of gender is being reexamined. People increasingly see family more fluidly as including both the bloodline we are born into and also the "family we choose" based on emotional affinity. Given the high value SK placed on tolerance and respect, and the strong stance he took against the inequities of the Indian caste system, I like to think that he would have embraced the liberalizing forces underlying all these changes, but that's not clear from the record.

> *Family life is a lot like using the bus service of India. A bus arrives at the station and is met by a great rush of people. It may have a capacity of fifty but over a hundred need to use it. If there is love in the family, everyone will be comfortable sitting close. They will think to themselves, "brother has important work to do here" and "sister must take care of business there," and patiently bear the pain of travelling together. The only way to ride this bus of family life is to take a seat deep in your heart. Doing that will change the direction of your whole life. This is what I am pointing out to you, that only by loving your family will you see the occasions to be patient and tolerant with everyone in society. Humankind is one family traveling together; that is the deepest truth.*

Danna and I never had children, a defining fact in our personal lives that limits my ability to address the full scope of issues pertinent to this chapter.[1] While lacking any experience of parenting, I have gained some understanding of the role of family on the path of yoga. All of us have a need for the feeling of belonging bestowed by good relationships with parents, children, and other relatives. To the extent it's possible to nurture those into caring and supportive relationships, it makes sense to do so. As you practice yoga, you will clarify your purpose and aims in life. The great majority of us will pursue these in the context of a nuclear family unit and extended clan. A harmonious family empowers its members to pursue their individual goals free from the aggravating friction of dissent and disapproval.

---

[1] I feel that it would be a great service to the yoga community for other householders to write about or otherwise share what they've learned about practicing yoga while parenting.

To foster this harmony, you must learn to value the well-being of your loved ones, and help in the collective effort to meet everyone's needs. Acting dynamically to accomplish your aims in life, while also enabling the success of others, is a challenging task, and one that will develop your character and personality. A person who learns these lessons at home can apply them outside in society to enjoy these benefits in the broader context of a supportive emotional surround. The inner peace and reduction in outer conflict this provides is a big aid in doing depth yoga practice, where the goal is to establish harmony with the cosmos and radiate love and light to the world. This is why in SK's thinking the quest for success and spiritual awakening starts with love in the family:

My definition of unbearable suffering is living in a household racked by enmity and quarrels, so I've always adapted my behavior to my family and loved ones. But I also never compromise those principles that I consider undeniably correct. For example, I have decided to pursue the path of yoga. This is my firm resolve and aim in life. So I must fulfill this aim, but do it in a way that my family and loved ones will be happy. Your purpose and goals in life may be different, but this is the hot fire that we all must pass through.

The pace of life has dramatically increased since Swami Kripalu's death in 1981. Riding the crest of a technological tsunami that is revolutionizing how we communicate and interact, society has grown painfully polarized. With members on opposite sides of widening political and other rifts, many families have fractured. I am not suggesting that we can go back to the simpler times and ways of village India. Yet these teachings can still speak to us today, provided we are willing to take them to heart.

A close disciple asked me about his students, "Who should be given mantra initiation? Who should be taught asana and pranayama? Who should be taught meditation? And what initiation should be given to one who has advanced beyond even these?" I told him to teach all his students love for the family. This requires us to become tolerant, learn to sacrifice, and gain humility. Humility only comes when we are quick to recognize the inhumility in ourselves and know how to remove it. Only by completing these lessons does the personality develop, after which the practice of yoga will be easy.

For a pair of teachings stories that link familial love and the spiritual life, see "The Women and Their Dearest Treasure" and "The Marriage of Divarka and Kalapata" in Appendix 2.

CHAPTER 16
THE IMPORTANCE OF CHARACTER BUILDING

Take up your abode in an ashram every now and then. Surrounded by other yogis, you'll find encouragement for your practice and many of the forces that commonly trouble the mind will be absent. Ashram living elevates your life by teaching you self-discipline, regular schedule, and how to fulfill your daily obligations as service. At first it is easy to be enthusiastic, but sustained yoga practice surfaces all kinds of problems so they can be resolved. Even at the ashram, you should expect to encounter difficulty.

Danna and I moved into Kripalu Center as ashram residents in 1989. For the better part of a decade, we'd taken programs, volunteered in various capacities, been initiated as disciples, and led a regional support group back home. There was no wishy-washiness in our decision to join the residential staff. We sold our house, then Danna's car, and quit our jobs. Packing a roomful of possessions in my Nissan pickup, we drove to the ashram and promptly sold the truck. Our last act as non-residents was to tithe the proceeds of the house sale to the yoga community we knew well, and in which we planned to spend the rest of our lives.

One reason we felt comfortable taking these seemingly rash actions was that the ashram was founded to promote the path of yoga taught by Swami Kripalu, upon which students and teachers alike practice character building to embody a high degree of personal integrity. Character building is the practical expression of the ethical principles applicable to all presented in chapter 7. The ashram was meant to reflect those values in action, and all its residents were expected to be actively involved in this process. The best way to illustrate how I came to understand the importance of SK's teachings on character building is to tell you a little about the ups and downs of our ashram experience, now so long ago.

In our first year of residency, Danna and I were housed separately. Our only alone time was Sunday afternoons, when long hikes through the Berkshire hills helped us catch up and mentally process all that was happening in our independent lives. As novice residents, we were ineligible for any cash allowance. Without income to pay my bar dues, I surrendered my license to practice law. Similarly, Danna had interrupted her string of successful library positions, aware that the resulting hole in her resume might jeopardize her chances of landing a future job. We made these sacrifices willingly, seeing them as part of what it meant to be members of a vowed religious order, knowing that many others had sacrificed similarly. It felt like we'd won the lottery when we finally got a twelve-by-twelve room and started receiving $35 a month to supplement the food and housing provided to us in-kind.

Thus began what we would come to call our honeymoon years in the ashram. For six months, I was assigned to the kitchen's scrub sink, washing the endless parade of dirty pots and pans produced by the cook's team, and keeping several industrial-sized steam kettles clean and perpetually ready to start the next meal. From there I was transferred to the resident business office, where I maintained the ashram's personnel files, signed on new staff members, disbursed the monthly cash allowance, engraved name tags and office door signs, and performed all sorts of one-off projects. I loved both of these roles, each of which kept me engaged and in high spirits.

After a year in the health for life office, Danna was assigned the role of room booker. Her job was to prioritize all the scheduling requests for program rooms and staff meeting spaces. She also kept the guest bulletin boards up to date by posting the locations of the daily yoga classes, workshop sessions, and other activities. From there she was moved into the educational resources department, where her librarian skills were helpful in indexing the ashram's archive of teachings. Alongside our mid-level administrative positions, we were members of the guest yoga team teaching a few classes a week. It was exciting to be part of a pioneering nonprofit bringing yoga to the world. Despite our limited time together, we were doing well as a couple, each of us enjoying a palpable sense of growth and forward movement in our individual lives.

A significant portion of my inquiry into Swami Kripalu's life and teaching legacy took place during this period, when I had easy access through Danna to a wealth of otherwise unavailable materials. Squinting to make out the words of a faint lecture transcript I was reading before bed in our tiny room, SK was saying that he wasn't afraid of death, which is a natural stage of the lifecycle everyone must face. But as a guru there was one thing he did fear: *the danger posed by a half-awakened disciple*. No explanation followed but the implication was clear. It worried him to have students in prominent teaching roles where their lack of spiritual maturity might position them to do harm. Unsure what to make of this statement, I turned off the light, oblivious that the cause for his trepidation would soon become apparent in the very place the two of us had dedicated ourselves to serving.

Near this time, I was abruptly transferred into the legal department and brought up to speed on a highly-confidential project. The guru's income had risen with the rapid growth of the guest center. No one could say how much he was making because his income was divided up between various departments. What was called his salary as the ashram's spiritual director came to him through normal accounting department channels. But there were also royalties paid by the retail shop for book and audio tape sales, and teaching honorariums paid by the programs department. Off the ashram's books entirely were revenue splits paid directly to him by outside seminar hosts, which I learned were tracked by the outreach department. There was concern that his overall income might be high enough to conflict with the ashram's nonprofit charter.

Once given the green light by the ashram higher ups, it was easy to get the numbers from the department heads and add them up. The total compensation figure raised my eyebrows—and Danna's when I shared it with her. That motivated us to spend a Sunday at Boston University's law library. Opening a nonprofit law finder, I looked under the heading "excessive compensation" and made a lengthy list of citations that started with L. Ron Hubbard of Scientology and ended with the televangelists Jim and Tammy Faye Bakker. In the finder's supplement, I found a reference to a recent case involving the CEO of United Way,

William Aramony, which had been in the news. Danna pulled the books from the shelves and piled them on the table next to me. Hours later we emerged from the stacks seriously shaken by the legal implications of what the IRS calls "benefits inuring." Everything we found indicated the guru's compensation was jeopardizing Kripalu Center's tax-exempt status and placing the entire ashram community at risk.

Monday dawned, and after morning yoga I relayed all this to my supervisor, who instructed me to go back to the department heads and get figures for the last five years. We used this data to plot his annual compensation on a graph, which made the steep upward slope of the trend line obvious. Something had to be done, as the situation was rapidly getting worse. My supervisor asked me to combine the legal research and compensation data into a memo and fax it to Kripalu Center's Washington-based tax attorney for review. The fax produced an immediate callback. At two-times the publicly-disclosed compensation of Billy Graham, America's foremost minister, the guru's pay rate was indefensible. As soon as possible, it needed to be cut in half to comply with IRS standards for religious leaders.

By sending out that memo under my name, I unwittingly became the point person of an administrative effort to slash the guru's salary. A year of hard work followed, but one entirely unlike my happy-go-lucky times in the kitchen and resident business office. Sworn to secrecy, this project was a shadowy, behind-the-scenes struggle that brought me and Danna into direct conflict with the guru and his second in command, a zealous woman devotee who wielded considerable power as the ashram's chief executive.

Formal legal opinions were solicited from two expert tax attorneys, who came to the ashram at considerable expense so the guru could question them. Following their lead, I drafted a new contract that capped the guru's total compensation at the upper limit of the allowable pay range, which could have been accepted quickly to document the organization's prompt resolution of this non-compliance. But only after a protracted negotiation that kept the status quo in place for another six months was it finally signed and put into place. Several tax years would have to elapse before Kripalu Center could pass an IRS audit, but a big step back from the cliff of legal calamity had been taken.

Once this work had been completed, there was no way that Danna and I could reconcile the guru's finances with the vow of simplicity taken by ashram residents, which I had personally administered in resident business. This was compounded by the attitude he privately displayed to us with regards to his own life, which was pragmatic and far less aspirational that his public persona. The dissonance became intolerable for us when he began making misleading statements in community gatherings to counter any rumors that might be circulating about his finances. While holding up renunciation as the ideal to which all ashram residents should aspire, the guru wasn't practicing what he preached, and he wasn't being truthful either.

Danna and I had maintained confidentiality and otherwise managed to keep our bearings through a difficult twelve months. But in the process, our ashram honeymoon came to a crushing end. We'd entered the community as true believers, intent on staying for life. But only four years later, we were out the door. We relocated around Danna, who landed a job cataloging books at the Salem Public Library in the Roanoke Valley of Virginia.

We had just moved into a fixer-upper house a few blocks from the library when we received a call from a close ashram friend. The entire community was reeling in shock and disbelief. Incontrovertible evidence had surfaced that the guru had sexual relations with several female students over many years, including a longstanding affair with the current chief executive. This was an egregious violation of the ashram's relationship guidelines under which the majority of residents were not only single but required to be celibate. Those unable to comply with the rules against persistent flirting let alone physical contact were routinely and often unceremoniously kicked out. In the wake of these sexual revelations, allegations were surfacing about other abuses of money and power. A scandalous storm was brewing, and our friend wanted us to know about it right away.

It was indeed a perfect storm, whose fury quickly extended beyond the parochial ashram community. Within a week, a feature story in the *Boston Globe* brought national media attention to bear upon Kripalu Center and its spiritual director. When statements made by the guru about the number of women involved proved fallacious, he was ousted by the ashram's board of trustees. Within a month, another of Swami Kripalu's American students was toppled from his ashram pedestal by similar revelations. Then came a visit by a respected member of our community who had moved to Kayavarohan, India a few years earlier to become a swami. She shared her story of being sexualized by SK's top student there. With none of his apparent successors left standing, everyone bore painful witness to the devastating effects of spiritual leaders falling prey to the unconscious forces of grandiosity, greed, and lust.

Leaving the ashram was like stepping out of a tight shoe for Danna. Happy in her new job, she shifted into a period of steady self-development that culminated a decade later in her emergence as a poet. But I struggled mightily, feeling aimless and unable to find meaningful work. Several months later, when the ashram asked me to rejoin its legal team on an hourly basis to help deal with the aftermath of the scandal, I jumped at the chance. Lawyering all day in my home office, I enrolled in Radford University and began taking night classes for a master's degree in counseling and human development. Ostensibly, I was broadening my career options. Deeper down, I was educating myself on cult dynamics and trying to make sense of my ashram experience.

The questions I was asking were not simple. Why had our ashram's guru, who was not by nature a bad person and had once been genuinely sincere and devoted, fallen so far short of yoga's ideals? Was there a lesson to be learned from his yoga practice gone awry? And what did the multiple scandals within our yoga lineage mean about Swami Kripalu's teachings on ethics and character building? Were they fatally flawed? If not, how had he avoided the pitfalls into which all of his top students and so many other westernized gurus plunged? I wanted to understand these issues in the light of western psychology. And not just for my own sake, but because an epidemic of teacher misconduct was affecting the American yoga movement and spiritual communities across the globe.

No one expects the leader of a social organization to be spotless in character. But anyone at the helm of a spiritual organization must by necessity be impeccable in their conduct. An ashram is a sovereign world unto itself. Its administration can only be handled by senior inmates of immaculate character steeped in its distinctive teachings and traditions. Many inhabitants of the surrounding region contribute to an ashram's sustenance. Taking retreat or refuge there, they come under its influence, and no harm of any kind should be felt by them as a result. A true spiritual leader must first be a great psychologist, as the path to pure conduct passes through all of the mental stages of character building. As a practicing yogi becomes more powerful, it is easy for them to grow egotistical. To think the body and mind are purified by a little progress is incorrect. Only by completing the process of character building does an aspirant arrive at a place of true humility. Only then can he or she serve as a genuine ambassador of yoga.

Kripalu Center's legal committee would labor long and hard to arrive at a settlement that not only compensated the five women who came forward as victims, but also provided some redress to the two hundred or so senior residents most impacted by the scandal. Admittedly, this was only the tip of a sizeable iceberg. The entire ashram community included nearly 5,000 members with many involved to a degree that left them feeling betrayed. Angry and disillusioned, some gave up entirely on the spiritual path. Worse yet, the shock waves from our ashram's downfall would ripple out in all directions and tarnish the positive image of yoga that everyone had worked to foster.

Situations like this are exceedingly complex. It's tempting to place the entirety of the blame upon the guru's shoulders, but certain members of his inner circle were also at fault. It can even be argued that the entire ashram community was complicit by surrounding the guru with adoring followers who mirrored back only his positive qualities, causing him to lose touch with reality. While there is plenty of blame to go around, that does not change the fact that the guru was the ashram's spiritual leader, and his moral and ethical lapses lie at the center of all this harm.

The blow struck by the guru's indiscretions would ultimately prove fatal to the already-unraveling ashram. Within a few short years, the residential community officially disbanded. The resulting diaspora scattered ashram residents across nearly all fifty states and various countries. Shortly after I completed my graduate studies, Danna and I returned to the Berkshires in 1998 to help with the start-up of the retreat center that eventually took the ashram's place. With the benefit of hindsight, I believe there are worthwhile answers to each of the questions posed above. But before they can be meaningfully discussed, I need to detail the process SK called *charitya vidhan*, which means "the process of forming a salutary character."

CHAPTER 17
CHARACTER BUILDING THROUGH PRACTICING THE OPPOSITE

It's easy to straighten out the tail of a dog, but the moment you let go it snaps back to its original shape. This shows why yoga places such great emphasis on character building. Consciously or unconsciously, each of us acts as prompted by our underlying character traits. Our actions reflect these traits, which in turn reveal our underlying intentions, whether helpful or hurtful. To be free to make our own happiness, we must learn how to dissolve the undesirable traits that cause us to behave in ways that bring us pain and are disagreeable to others, even though that is not our conscious intent.

Character building is a topic so seldom addressed in yoga circles that a reader might assume it originated with Swami Kripalu. But that would be a mistake. The Yoga Sutra codified the core of this time-honored technique in a single verse: When the mind is disturbed by vices and thoughts contrary to yoga, their opposites should be cultivated. (II.33) While the idea expressed in this pithy aphorism is clear, it's not readily apparent how to put it into practice. That's where SK was inventive. His commentary provides the conceptual framework needed to apply this teaching effectively in life. He begins his instruction with an overview of the technique that includes a plausible explanation of how it originated:

Do not wrestle with a fault that you want to remove. Wrestling only increases the disturbance of the mind, allowing the excited fault to lift you up and slam you to the ground. Unable to pull yourself up to fight again, you will eventually give up the battle forever. The best way to remove a fault is to dwell upon its opposite virtue. The ancient sages developed this practice, which they called the method of thinking the contrary (pratipaksha bhavanam). First, they noticed that the mind is able to think in one way, and think in the opposite way too. Then they saw that it is actually the nature of the mind to do this, to look at both sides of a pair of opposites and ask, "Which one of these two alternatives is better for me to select?" Discovering this, the sages quickly learned that people easily give up a harmful course of action when they are sufficiently impressed by advantageous thoughts of its opposite. Only after the import of this mental mechanism is understood does practicing the yogic virtues really become possible.

He goes on to chart out the step-by-step method. The first step is to make a commitment to keep your attention focused squarely on your own character, as the tendency to look outside and engage in what SK called *fault finding* is inimical to the type of one-pointed introspection that sparks self-development. Once this commitment is made, subsequent steps can be taken, but the habit of criticizing others to bolster your prevailing sense of self is strong. A practitioner should expect to reaffirm this non-judgmental stance many times before it is replaced by a natural inclination to engage in the remaining steps of the character building process.

I have gleaned many principles of character building from scriptures, the company of saints, the biographies of great men and women, and from my own experiences. Here I will describe only the foremost principle, which is that an aspirant should firmly decide: "I want to look only at my character." Why this exclusive focus? Because dwelling on the faults of others blocks you from seeing your own shortcomings. An eye keen to spot the faults of others is very ordinary and of no help to a yogi. The sharp inner vision able to view your own faults objectively is extraordinary and of great value. But to obtain it, you have to exert yourself and suffer a bit too. To practice character building, you must sincerely want to remedy your faults and increase your good qualities. Until that determination arises, objective self-seeing is not possible.

The next step is to survey the cornucopia of virtuous qualities that yoga sees as native to every soul. This preliminary study is what paves the way for an impactful character-building practice. Where the Yoga Sutra prescribes five restraints and five observances, SK drew from the full library of yogic texts to arrive at a comprehensive list of twenty-three virtues. Together these qualities represent yoga's attempt to catalog the positive attributes naturally displayed by a spiritually-awake person. Readers wanting to engage in this study are directed to the appendix of Character Building Principles for a distillation of how SK defined and taught each one.

> *Every yoga student knows the short-list of ethical precepts prescribed by Patanjali. But there are many other virtues praised in the yogic scriptures including faith, enthusiasm, courage, tolerance, compassion, patience, determination, discernment, self-confidence, right speech, charity, straightforwardness, steadfastness, humility, moderation in diet, consistent study of the doctrines, not overworking, refraining from excessive or obsessive spiritual practice, good company, peacefulness and inner quiet, learning to enjoy solitude, worshipping the sacred, and direct knowledge of the essence. Familiarize yourself with these virtues to gain an accurate picture of the soul's divine nature. Even though this picture can only be seen with the eyes of imagination, it is a great aid in the process of character building and the sure means to awaken qualities that would otherwise remain dormant and unknown. But one cannot grow spiritually merely by studying lists. For that, one must contemplate these qualities daily and act to bring them into expression.*

Most of us have an impoverished view of our Self or soul, which yoga teaches is overflowing with life energy, goodwill, and creative potential. From the viewpoint of yoga, the soul (atman) is a vast spiritual reservoir always ready to channel more of itself through the relatively small spigot of our body-mind. Each yogic virtue reflects a distinct facet of the soul's promise, and expressing it in action stirs the soul to greater aliveness. Studying these qualities reminds a student of the basic yogic approach. An adept yogi is not someone who has mastered each of these virtues one-by-one through willpower and discipline. Instead, a yogi utilizes the techniques of yoga to tap into the soul, which is precocious and already replete with them.

An ordinary person is blind to the divine nature of his own soul. Yoga considers this ignorance the primary cause of all the complicated problems we face in life. A glimmer of the soul's greatness can be seen in artists, athletes, and geniuses in all fields, each of whom has succeeded in re-awakening some aspect of the soul's slumbering intelligence. In most instances, these capacities have come forth through their unknowing practice of yoga-like principles, which has partially awakened their dormant soul power. At first, such an awakening reinvigorates the basic human capacities such as physical strength, willpower, logical thinking, accurate memory, and creative imagination. Many divine qualities follow including enthusiasm, courage, peace, happiness, joy, tolerance, forgiveness, charity, and mercy. All these qualities reflect not an individual's greatness, but the intelligence and pure responsiveness of the soul itself. A yogi able to access the soul gives up old ways easily as these divine predilections spontaneously come forth. For something to truly be yoga, it must aim to reawaken the consciousness of the soul.

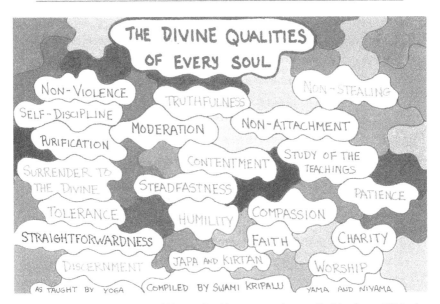

These are the 23 virtuous qualities praised by yoga and compiled by Swami Kripalu. Artwork by Danna Faulds.

THE CORE OF THE PRACTICE

The stage has now been set for character building to begin in earnest. Having surveyed the yogic virtues, find some way to keep them alive in your awareness. You may recall from chapter 7 that I hung a framed list of the restraints and observances in our yoga room, which I read each morning before exiting. As you go through your days, watch your behavior. Whenever you spot a shortcoming or come face-to-face with an obvious deficit in your character, affirm the opposite virtue. You are likely to find yourself returning to SK's commentary on the yogic virtues, as reflecting upon these and similar teachings can be trusted to keep you inspired, alert to the process, and progressing in the right direction.

While doing this practice of self-observation, clear patterns will emerge in your conduct, and the personal work you need to strengthen your character will come into view. Don't try to tackle all the yogic virtues at once. Any such attempt will only leave you feeling overwhelmed and defeated. Instead, bring all of your focus to bear upon a single principle as reflected in a specific facet of your character. The incremental shifts that result will add up to real change.

If you eat improperly, your stomach will hurt. In the same way, any time you violate a true character building principle, it will bring pain to some part of your system. While it's good to have heard all the principles, you can only work on one at a time. Find the area of your life that is causing you the most pain, and decide to place your attention there. Remain focused on that painful area, following it very closely, until you identify the positive movement that is needed to restore rightness and ease. In my simple example, to remedy indigestion it may be necessary to eat differently or adopt some form of exercise. Through self-observation and this kind of in-depth reflection, the solution to every problem can be found.

Unless you are willing to face your character defects, you will not find the answers you need to grow. You may stretch your body, close your eyes, and even control your breath, but if you avoid doing this self-analysis your progress on the path of yoga will be limited. This is of extreme importance, as a single bad habit may reduce a person to a sorry state while a single good habit may raise a person lost in misery to the status of a great man or woman. I am giving you a hundred pounds of guidance here. If you practice even a few ounces of it, that will be enough.

This was the focus of SK's yoga practice for what I call "his householder years," which carried over into his first decade as a monk.[1] Early each morning, he performed his yoga routines to stay spiritually attuned. While working as a music teacher or serving the villagers as a novice swami, he carefully observed his thoughts and actions. Sometime during the day, he found time for the vigorous exercise he needed to keep fit. Every evening before going to bed, he contemplated his daily interactions, using them as a mirror in which he could see his character reflected back to him. Contrasting his conduct with the vision of the soul espoused by the yogic scriptures, he earnestly strove to become a person of genuine goodwill.

It is impossible to not make mistakes in life. Difficult situations arise and knowingly or unknowingly we all take missteps. We don't realize that these mountains of mistakes are precisely where the springs of self-knowledge can begin to flow. Whenever I behave improperly during the day and am not able to see my error, the mistake will come looking for me during my evening introspection and say, "This is where you were at fault." Whenever such a mistake appears to me so clearly, I consider it a wonderful boon, as it helps me not make the same mistake again.

In the practice of character building, even a slanderous enemy can be an ally, as faults which have not been found after deep contemplation rise to the surface in the words of harsh critics. That is why the scriptures say that we should thank any person who helps us see our shortcomings. Speaking about this is easy, but to bear the insults required to practice it is very difficult. Yet anyone who grows to excel in life is by necessity wedded to the disciplines

---

[1] SK never married, but for ten years practiced yoga while working as a playwright and music teacher to support his mother and brother. For more on SK's practice of character building during this stage of his life, see chapters 3-5 of *Dharma Then Moksha*.

of self-observation and self-analysis. Practice them and you will also be successful.

This method of character building reminded me of the so-called "Prayer of Saint Francis," an anonymous writing that first appeared in an obscure French magazine in 1912 but is often attributed the Italian mystic and friar who lived from 1181 to 1226:

> Lord, make me an instrument of your peace: where there is hatred, let me sow love; where there is injury, pardon; where there is doubt, faith; where there is despair, hope; where there is darkness, light; where there is sadness, joy. O divine Master, grant that I may not so much seek to be consoled as to console, to be understood as to understand, to be loved as to love. For it is in giving that we receive, it is in pardoning that we are pardoned, and it is in dying that we are born to eternal life.

Recognizing the principle of sowing the opposite enshrined in this world-renowned prayer made me appreciate the universality of yoga's approach to character building. Saints are often credited for helping individuals in desperate straits to bring forth whatever soulful quality is needed to ease their difficulties. Before gaining this ability, it makes sense they would have to do this work for themselves. It felt like SK's method of character building was showing me how the libertine son of a silk merchant could become the spiritual benefactor we know as Saint Francis of Assisi.

A STUMBLING BLOCK TO ANTICIPATE

Through his personal practice and the experience he gained vicariously by instructing others, SK learned that the process of character building unfolds in a predictable manner. This enabled him to warn students of a significant roadblock they should expect to encounter. A new practitioner who starts to see their faults is often overwhelmed by feelings of guilt and shame. This is an early phase of the practice that must be seen for what it is—an indicator of progress—to enable the emotional pain associated with it to be tolerated before later and more objective phases of self-seeing can dawn.

> *The practice of yoga and self-observation purifies the mind, making it steady and mirror-like. But a seeker must remember that mirrors are of many types. In some mirrors, you see yourself smaller or bigger than you are. Only a perfect mirror gives you a true picture of yourself.*
>
> *At first, due to our self-centeredness, we will not be able to see our faults. We will look at an unreal picture of ourselves in a mirror that hides shortcomings from our sight. As we continue to practice, we gain the ability to see our faults and lower qualities. For a time, these loom large in the distorted mirror of the mind, which is why self-examination is always done with love. We must bear the pain of this stage, understanding that once we've seen our faults, we've accomplished the hardest part. We're a success, even though we may feel like a failure, because the fountain of self-knowledge is springing up in our heart.*
>
> *Gradually we begin to recognize that there are good qualities also. This starts another stage, in which we let go of lower qualities as higher qualities come in and keep increasing. Then we begin to see the good qualities in others too. All of these character building stages are part of our spiritual progress.*

Right from the start, it's helpful to know where this method is intended to carry you. While SK championed external accomplishment in many areas of life, he did not subscribe to that line of thinking when it comes to character building. Without a doubt, the practice of character building will bring you tangible benefits. It will raise your self-awareness by enabling you to see both your strengths and weaknesses. It will teach you to accept yourself, warts and all, and help you persist in the good conduct needed to bring your best self forward. Continued practice will make you more ethically-minded, and help you appreciate the practical value of high ideals. But any yoga practitioner who finds themselves feeling morally superior or touting their ethical integrity should realize they have taken a wrong turn into a dangerous cul-de-sac. The end goal of character building is not self-righteousness, or a smug sense of accomplishment, but humility.

> *A person who cannot see their own shortcomings is blind. But a person remains handicapped if they see their faults and do not know how to get rid of them by acquiring the opposite virtue. It is only the person who has grown strong by practicing character building to the limit of their capacity who finds their abode in humility.*
>
> *The idea that spiritual growth gives birth to pride is false. The branches of a tree laden with fruit bend low. A full vessel tips its head so the empty vessel can be filled. A mother stoops to lift her child. Where an egotistical person cannot keep from exhibiting their accomplishments in an attempt to puff up their self-image, a humble person makes little of their virtues and looks with compassionate eyes to the needs of others. They enjoy a sublime simplicity in which their good character is protected because thoughts of their own greatness never arise.*
>
> *When can it be said that an aspirant is fit to practice depth meditation? Only when they humbly recognize they have shortcomings, are willing to look at them carefully, find out the reasons for them, and sincerely work to remove their causes. This train of character building has many stops. You do not have to know in advance how it will get you to the final destination. If you board the train, it can be trusted to run on its rails. Just make sure your ticket gets punched to "humility" or you may end up at the wrong station.*

A FINAL STEP

After sustaining this practice for a number of years, a seasoned student can proceed to the final step of SK's methodical approach to character building. Choose a single virtue that deeply resonates with your purpose and outlook on life. Let the long list of yogic virtues recede into the background of your mind, as you practice this one with the intention to embody it completely.

> *Yoga practice exposes all our faults—that is its purpose. A devoted yogi bows before their altar each day and offers these faults to God.*

For a long time, there is a need for the constant application of the character-building technique. After that, what remains to be done by us?

All of the yogic virtues are intimately related with one another. A practitioner who fully develops a single virtue will procure every other one too. These virtues reflect the divine qualities of the soul. To be possessed by any one of them brings one's divinity forth. That is why it is said, "By grasping one flower of a garland, the whole garland of flowers is lifted." This saying guides us to take up the practice of a single virtue and keep it steady in our memory all the time.

A virtuous character is the best and most sublime of all accomplishments, but many subtle impurities will remain even after this step has been taken. That is why the Upanishads say: "The process of purifying the unclean mind is only completed in samadhi." This teaches us that a humble aspirant should continue to patiently ascend the ladder of yoga in order to attain direct knowledge of the soul.

SK never described himself as having progressed to the final step of character building. But I believe the record shows the single yogic virtue he chose to practice:

I consider straightforwardness supreme among the virtues. Its scriptural definition sounds simple: "to reveal our thoughts and feelings as they are, concealing nothing." But as people we play mind games to impress, fool, and mislead others. We cloak our crookedness in all sorts of guises to get what we want. Where crookedness gives birth to various forms of deceit, straightforwardness is the mother of all the other virtues. One who abandons crookedness in favor of straightforwardness becomes very direct, honest, and fit for meditation. Everyone considers themselves to be straightforward, but this is a pervasive delusion. It is more accurate to say that one hundred out of one hundred people are mistaken in measuring their own straightforwardness. And since I consider myself to be straightforward, I am one of the deluded ones.

RECAPPING THE METHOD

Everyone seems to agree on the formative role character plays in shaping our lives. The Greek sage Heraclitus may have been the first to express the idea that "character becomes destiny," but he was far from the last. Buddha echoes it in the Dhammapada: "All that we are arises with our thoughts. Speak or act with an impure mind, and trouble will follow you as the wheel follows the ox that draws the cart. Speak or act with a pure mind, and happiness will follow you as your shadow, unshakable." The New Testament book of Galatians says it this way in chapter 6: "Whatsoever a man soweth he shall also reap." These ancient ideas reverberate in the more current wording of Frank Outlaw, a successful American supermarket entrepreneur, that appears frequently online: "Watch your thoughts, they become words. Watch your words, they become actions. Watch your actions, they become habits. Watch your habits, they become character. Watch your character, for it becomes your destiny." While many affirm this idea, hardly anyone says how to apply it in life.

Here's a summary of SK's step-by-step approach to character building:

- Commit to looking only at your own character.
- Survey the "values of the soul" to familiarize yourself with the breadth of positive character traits that you already possess in seed form and are endeavoring to bring forth.
- Practice self-observation, seeing your shortcomings with an attitude of self-acceptance and love.
- Respond by mentally affirming and practicing the opposite virtue.
- Be sure to also acknowledge your good qualities.
- Work with a single virtue at a time, being content to make incremental progress.
- Cultivate patience, persisting in this technique for a long time, during which you learn to enjoy the character-building process.
- Pick one virtue that resonates deeply with your perspective on life, practicing intensively to embody it fully.
- Continue your on-the-mat yoga and meditation practice.

Ultimately, Swami Kripalu taught that when you boil the spiritual life down to its essence, you find that all contemplative techniques are designed to facilitate what he called *self-observation without judgment*. Much of his practical instruction on character building was delivered under this catchy rubric, which describes how a person able to witness their faults will find them withering away:

> *I observed silence while practicing yoga for eighteen years. What benefit did I get? Rather than listing all the benefits, I will give you the most useful secret silence enabled me to discover. While doing yoga, your mind will grow increasingly subject to your control. Use this growth to allow a portion of your awareness to remain a witness as you perform your actions in life. By doing this practice, you will see that the witness is always there, even when the mind is greatly disturbed, if you can keep a wakeful attitude. It is this ability to see yourself in all mind states that catalyzes self-analysis and becomes the foundation for spiritual progress.*
>
> *Remain neutral and objective. Be like a movie camera whose impressionable film catches all the movements going on around it. To whatever extent you are able observe the subtle movements of the mind in your self-observation, to that extent faults will wither away and you will receive the light of consciousness. At first, you will only skim across the surface of the mind. Then you will begin to observe with depth and pick up detail. If you do self-observation properly, you will never see the faults of others, as your attention will always be on yourself. That is the sign that true self-observation is occurring. Self-observation without judgment is the highest spiritual practice. Whatever you seek in life can be found through it. Its persistent practice will enable you to master your mind and ego, carrying you all the way to the threshold of samadhi.*

For instructions on how to practice his technique of self-observation contemplatively, see the "Witness Meditation" in Appendix 3.

BE A DISCERNING STUDENT

A dutiful student does as directed. But a discerning one also asks the hard questions, like those posed at the close of the last chapter: Why had our ashram's guru fallen so far short of yoga's ideals? Is there a lesson for me to learn from his yoga gone awry? And what do the multiple scandals among SK's top students mean about his teachings on character building? Are they fatally flawed? How had SK avoided the ethical pitfalls into which all of his top students and so many other westernized gurus plunged?

It goes without saying that these issues are enormously complex. But I believe a few points can be made that are worth sharing. All of his top students began practicing potent forms of energy-raising yoga earlier in their growth process than SK, and before they had developed their characters to the stage of humility. As a result, they were unable to channel the entirety of their amplified energy into healthy outlets and selfless works. Instead, the excess drove each to eventually succumb to some form of arrogance that was acted out in unethical behaviors.

Upon meeting SK, I immediately saw that he displayed two seemingly opposite qualities. He radiated great spiritual power, while displaying a child-like innocence and warmth. It was this remarkable mix of strength and sensitivity that enabled him to identify with others, genuinely care about their well-being, and effectively guide them. I believe it was these kind of character traits that safeguarded him from scandal. Perhaps his top students tasted the power that comes with high-energy yoga too early and never attained the high degree of humility required to balance out the equation?[2]

The aim of a student setting out on the path of yoga is growth, self-knowledge, and the realization of God. Sincere and accomplished students are likely to assume the position of a spiritual teacher. If many people are attracted to such a student-guru by virtue of their disciplined conduct, genuine progress, and energetic charisma, that purity of purpose is easily lost. If mass popularity results, it often leads to deceit, pride, and false shows of humility. Accepting the exaggerated status of master, the purity of the

---

[2] SK was outspoken about the difficulty of honoring ethics while doing yoga practices designed to rouse primal energies and set powerful unconscious forces into motion. These practices are known to greatly intensify what Western philosophy calls "the passions." This is why he chose to live the second half of his life in seclusion. Discussion of this important topic is continued in the next book in this series and specifically the chapter titled "Kundalini in Practice."

student is forever lost. Misled by the ego, they reject the need for continued practice and divert the power meant for samadhi to gratify their material desires for wealth, pleasure, and position in society. This is how the path that was meant to open a gateway to divine experience erodes the character and becomes a doorway to downfall.

The difference between SK's character and that of his top students was apparent to many of his followers. None of them could really fill his shoes after his death in 1981. This is why, in my opinion, he has no true successor. The scandals that engulfed all those positioned to succeed him only confirmed this, in a sad and painful way.

While trying to answer these questions for myself, I was aided by the work of Ken Wilber, who makes an interesting point. While enlightened in many ways, the spiritual traditions were largely unaware of the dynamic of repression, which was only explained in the twentieth century by modern psychology. Many forms of traditional meditative practice instruct a student to "dis-identify" from the body and mind, which allows these "disowned" emotions to accumulate outside the view of the conscious mind. There they become part of what psychology calls "the shadow" and get unconsciously acted out when opportunities present. In clinical treatment, psychotherapy takes an opposite approach to yoga by encouraging a client to own these emotions by giving them a voice, and then either working them through inwardly or expressing them outwardly via healthy outlets.

After hearing Wilber state this view, I was astonished to find places in SK's writings that indicate he was well aware of this phenomenon:

According to Sigmund Freud, the unconscious mind is the residence of many repressed desires. These remain latent and only come forth when the right conditions present. Even as they are being symbolically expressed in dreams or acted out in real life, the conscious mind remains ignorant of its unconscious motives. The identity of the repressed desire is kept hidden from the conscious mind. This censoring enables the unconscious mind to run whichever way it wants in search of gratification. That is how repressed desires and unconscious behaviors create havoc in our lives. A fully realized yogi is one who has seen that they are the sum total of all these conscious and

> *unconscious energies—which means they have completely awakened and there is no more falling down into unconscious actions. Until then, there is every possibility that a yogi's conduct may be motivated by selfishness and falsehood.*

I believe SK's emphasis on character building arises from an unavoidable truth of human nature. Unless and until our faculties are firmly grounded in humility and perfect Self-knowledge has been gained, they are apt to be misused. This is writ large in the multitude of spiritual teachers and gurus who preach celibacy or monogamy while having extramarital affairs, and extol the virtue of renunciation and material sacrifice while hoarding money. But it would be duplicitous of me to be throw stones in their direction. When placed in a top position of organizational leadership, I quickly fell off my ethical high horse too.[3] After asking the hard questions, discerning students do not get sidetracked for long. They regain their bearings and return to the foremost principle: Keep your focus squarely on your own character!

APPLYING THIS CHAPTER IN PRACTICE

While studying SK's lectures on character building, I ran into differing guidance on the mindset he recommended for practitioners. In some places, he spoke convincingly of the paramount role of self-discipline:

> *In the process of purifying the character, a resolute will is of primary significance. The power of will is synonymous with the power of the Self. Self-possessed will has an indomitable, rocklike power that can fend off detrimental elements through its unflinching determination. At the same time, it imperceptibly marshals all the mind's positive qualities to create circumstances conducive to overcoming difficulties. Thus, it can be said that resolute willpower is the foundation upon which one's personality flourishes and gets refined and embellished. With burning idealism, an aspirant must drive the pole of decisiveness deeply into the ground of their life, as*

---

[3] This story is told in Danna's memoir, *Into the Heart of Yoga*.

> the task of purifying one's character and personality is so arduous that it can never be accomplished otherwise.

In other places, he advocated an almost mirror-image approach of relying on surrender and grace:

> *I am not a great believer in courage. The average person is scared to death of all that's required to develop the qualities of good character needed to put us on the road to a higher level of self-expression and success. Some of us are a little bolder and imagine we can do it. But one-hundred percent of us will reach a crisis on the way to becoming an ideal human being and discover that we don't have a single drop of courage left to go one step further.*
>
> *By all means, exert yourself to rid your mind of bad thoughts. And do only good actions. But you can keep doing this forever and it will not bring you any closer to perfection. You may plan it all out. You may act to strengthen your resolve. But the way of willpower alone never works. It is only by opening yourself to the soul force flowing from within that the divine power of thinking, the divine power of creativity, and all of the other divine qualities can emerge. This is the only way through which a human can arrive at a genuine sense of self-mastery and realize a purity of mind that otherwise remains beyond comprehension. I may not be a great believer in courage, but I am a great believer in God's benevolence, whose way of grace is always granted. We may start boldly and proceed from there, but eventually we must surrender to grace.*

While these teachings appear contradictory, a student must remember that character building is a long-term endeavor. I've come to see that these two mindsets speak to different stages of the process. At first, a resolute will is required to start and persist in the effort. In the middle, a mix of willfulness and surrender is needed to sustain progress. Near the end, willful effort must be allowed to fall away for a long-term practitioner who has gained a measure of humility to let go into the flow of a larger intelligence.

It's likely that SK would deny that there is anything original in his character building teachings. He'd probably point back with reverence to sage Patanjali and the long line of yogis who came before him. But after reading countless books and scriptures, I disagree. In my experience, the manner in which he links moral and ethical development to mystical yoga is unique. Typically, these two elements of yoga practice are treated as if they exist in entirely different domains. Not so in SK's approach, where good character is an integral factor in spiritual awakening:

> *The soul is infinite and difficult to comprehend. As a result, the science of yoga is misunderstood. In the view of yoga, a human being is an instrument of the divine soul existing in the world. As the sun does not need to come down from the sky to give light, so the soul does not need to wander into a village or city. It can do its work indirectly through a person of good character.*
>
> *Through the science of yoga, a yogic saint purifies their character. The humility that results enables them to bow easily to the promptings of the soul, which is why such men and women are credited with inspiring good works and even propagating miracles. Not understanding this, people flock to them as miracle workers and do not value the techniques of character building.*
>
> *In the science of yoga, all divine works and miracles are seen to originate from the soul or God, and not from the personality of any particular human being. It must always be remembered that the greatest power granted by yoga is direct spiritual knowledge of the soul and its divine union with God, the receipt of which has a special perquisite, a virtuous character full of loving humbleness.*

For a teaching story that affirms the importance of character buildings foremost principle, see "The Nature of a Yogi" in Appendix 2.

CHAPTER 18
MANTRA YOGA

It is not easy to grasp how all the benefits promised in the yogic texts can come about by repeating a mantra over and over. One can resolve this mystery only through experience. As practiced initially, mantra recitation increases the ability to focus awareness and direct the attention. It is by applying this mental focus in the subsequent stages of practice that all these benefits can be attained. But an in-depth understanding of its theory and technique is required for mantra yoga to be done correctly and deliver on its promises.

You may be surprised to learn that relatively few of Swami Kripalu's Indian students routinely practiced asana and pranayama. Most of them stayed focused on the four practices he emphasized for householders: healthy lifestyle, character building, karma yoga, and mantra yoga.[1] It was relatively late in SK's life—during the 1960s and '70s—when he encountered a cohort of Westerners eager to learn hatha yoga and use its body-based techniques to grow spiritually. It was primarily in response to them that he began recommending the practice of asana and pranayama to non-renunciates.

---

[1] To be clear, SK did encourage asana and pranayama practice to develop *virya raksha*, a state of virility traditional associated with manliness and heroism. But he saw this high degree of bodily strength and energetic effervescence as only essential for hatha and tantric yogis whose progress depended upon it. The foundational on-the-mat practice he emphasized for students living active lives in society, especially during his primary years of teaching, was mantra yoga. Karma yoga—the practice of skillfully discharging one's duties in life with an attitude of service to others—is addressed in chapter 21.

None of this should be taken to mean that his Indian householder students weren't devoted yogis. It's just the path up the proverbial mountain of yoga that most of them chose utilized the view and practice of mantra yoga as presented in this chapter.

> *Among the yogas, mantra yoga is most ancient. Each of the four Vedas has a section devoted exclusively to the use of mantras. Many yoga schools offer a method enabling students to attain all four aims of life, but mantra yoga is unique among them because it can be practiced by anyone from the most-lowly to the most-high. To some extent, everyone is acquainted with the power of sound. A thunderous rainstorm shakes and scares us. The sweet tones of a musical instrument enchant the mind and delight us. The crying or laughing of a loved one makes us feel sad or joyful. But these are ordinary forms of sound power. An adept mantra yogi knows that sound power also has an extraordinary form called nada. Many teachers dispense mantras, but fail to provide the guidance necessary for their effective practice. I know this from experience. Through the religious training provided me by my parents, I developed a love for mantras and chanted them from childhood. But only after practicing at the feet of my beloved Gurudev and receiving his pure instruction did the practice of mantra begin to flourish in me. Now I will try to tell you how to unlock the energy hidden in these scientific sound formulas called mantras.*

NADA: THE PRIMORDIAL SOUND CURRENT

The keystone concept in this view is conveyed by the Sanskrit word nada (pronounced nad), which means "the primordial sound current." In mantra yoga, all of existence is seen as coming into being through a rich mix of vibratory emanations perpetually sounding forth from an unseen and silent spiritual source. While described as a sound to make the concept clear and relatable, the yogis knew that nada was not a sonic phenomenon. Sound waves pass through the medium of air, a known material element in their system of metaphysics. They described nada as emanating from a subtler realm called ether.

> *The root of every mantra is subtle sound or nada. It is through the activity of this subtle sound that all the objects and elements of nature arose and evolved. This includes the audible sounds, syllables, letters, words, and sentences of human language and music. But the yogis knew that nada was much more subtle than sound. Nada was seen to flow through the element of ether, which is finer than earth, water, fire, air, or space. Beyond ether is only Brahman, the Supreme source.*

The concept of nada is closely linked to the broader notion that the material universe arises from an "eternal cosmic vibration" signified by the syllable Om or Aum. This ancient Vedic idea is woven into all the major Indian religions—Hinduism, Buddhism, Jainism, and Sikhism.[2] In these traditions, the Om vibration is believed to undergird and pervade the universe.

> *Om is the best sound formula of all, which is why it is called the sacred syllable. When chanted or meditatively uttered, it causes you to spontaneously close your eyes and gaze upward to see the inner light and sense what lies beyond it. When heard as an inner sound, it captures the attention, making the mind one-pointed and carrying you beyond all sound. It is into this inner silence that the outer world dissolves. It is here that a yogi can distinguish between what is perishable (the body-mind) and what is imperishable (the atman or soul) and resituate the identity in its true form (shift into Self-realization).*

Being integral parts of creation, this cosmic vibration resonates deep within us. All the techniques of mantra yoga are meant to attune and

---

[2] Citing the Mandukya Upanishad, mythologist Joseph Campbell says; "Om is a word that represents to our ears the sound of the energy of the universe of which all things are manifestations." Nada plays a prominent role in the Sikh religion and its yoga, where it is called *shabd*. In common religious usage, shabd means the word as in the basis for human speech. Esoterically, shabd is the sound current vibrating within our being that can be meditated upon to discover our direct energetic connection to God. Contemporary yoga includes many names and variations of inner sound meditation.

harmonize our bodies and minds with different frequencies of this subtle vibratory energy. While the vibration itself is beyond the range of human hearing, yoga teaches that an auditory expression of it can be perceived in depth meditation. For those who gain the ability to hear and meditate upon inner sound, it becomes a dynamic focal point that can be consciously followed back to experience the silent spiritual source from which it is always emanating.

Many of the world religions have teachings that parallel those of mantra yoga. Christianity says, "In the beginning was the Word, and the Word was with God." This suggests the entire universe was spoken into existence. A yogi treats the Word with equal reverence and calls it the pranav mantra or Om. The masters of mantra yoga consider Om to be the seed from which the universe sprouted and is continually sustained. In their minds, this whole world is composed of nothing but subtle sound vibrations. Without the divine utterance, there would be no cosmos, no human existence, no words, no musical notes or songs, and no dance of creation.

The yogic concepts of Om and nada are consistent but not identical. Om is a relatively simple description of how the universe came into being that meshes well with the practice of yogic meditation. A multitude of yoga schools subscribe to this view. Nada is a more nuanced teaching tailored to the practice of mantra yoga in which the primordial Om gives birth to a cosmic symphony of vibratory energies, octaval tones, and modulating wave frequencies that reflect the vast diversity of the material universe in which we live. Every aspect of existence—including all the different forms of life—are seen to have a signature sound formula or mantra that resonates with its unique vibration and constitutes its true name. You might think that mantra yoga's only purpose is developing the ability to hear the inner Om sound and discovering what lies behind it. But mantra yoga has too many other applications for that to be accurate. It is better to think of mantra yoga as learning to speak the language of mantra in all sorts of beneficial ways.

What is nada? Where does it come from? What can it be used for? The purpose of this long discussion has been to examine these questions. Now I will summarize. Yoga tells us that nada is the subtle energy from which this material world has come into form and into which it can be dissolved to realize its spiritual source. We're also told that we can become reacquainted with this nada by meditating upon the subtlest sound that can be found within our range of hearing.

It is difficult to understand where nada comes from until it's experienced directly. But having an accurate conception is an aid to practice, so I will simplify. What's beyond visibility becomes spiritual light (jyoti), which becomes love-filled sound (nada), which becomes everything in creation (prakriti). Your Bible says, "the Word became flesh." In receiving divine messages, all of humanity's highest saints have realized that God's speech is the vehicle of creation. They called it the language of truth, the divine language, or the language without any pollution. In India, this is the language of mantra, whose sound formulas are not meaningless combinations of letters and words. They are potent expressions of nada that have many uses.

Meditatively reciting these mantras has an intoxicating effect on the mind that causes the thought waves to fall into a harmonizing rhythm. All sorts of good qualities and conditions can be made manifest by this attunement practice that yoga calls nada nusandhana (fixing one's attention first on the mantra and eventually on inner sound). Based on these ideas is a method of practice through which one can progress all the way to moksha, which is why among mantra yogis these teachings on nada are given the highest importance.

We will return to the view and theories of mantra yoga in the next chapter. In practice, few of us can quiet the mind sufficiently to hear the inner sound without a course of methodical training. In mantra yoga, that training begins with the practice of mantra japa.

MANTRA JAPA

The Sanskrit word *japa* literally means "to mutter." In yoga, japa is the persistent recitation of a mantra to establish its sound and meaning deep in the psyche. The mantra can be spoken out loud in a normal voice, said in a quiet whisper that is simultaneously vocalized and listened to in order to command one's full attention, or repeated silently within the practitioner's mind. It can also be musically chanted. When recited in a sitting posture as a contemplative practice, it is often performed with the help of a japa mala, a string of 108 beads used to track the number of recitations. The mala plays another important role, as fingering the beads provides a tactile sensation that helps a practitioner stay present and anchored in their body.[3]

The mechanics of mantra japa can easily be learned online, where all sorts of instructive videos are available. During our initiation ceremony, Danna and I were taught a three-step technique based on Swami Kripalu's teachings. First the mantra is recited aloud in a steady voice for a few minutes. This active technique is called *vaikhar japa*, and it helps beginners shut out distractions. Next comes a period of *upamshu japa*, in which the mantra is intoned in a soft and heartfelt whisper to ignite devotion. When the awareness has grown internalized, a practitioner moves into *manisika japa*, the silent recitation of the mantra in the mind. This is the most difficult form of japa in which to sustain focus, as it's easy for the mind to wander off into daydreams or problem solving. But if concentration can be sustained, this inward recitation is considered to have the strongest impact.

After a period of practicing this three-step japa technique, it becomes easy to sit down and move smoothly into inward recitation without spending much—or any—time in out loud or whispered recitation. The focused and sustained inward recitation of mantra is meant to naturally bring the mind into silence, which is a cue to end japa and begin meditation.

A practitioner of mantra japa should know that reciting a mantra is not nearly as simple as it seems. All the letters in our alphabets, and each of the words in our vocabulary, are rooted in the cosmic nada. To speak a word, we must first recall it in our mind. Before the sound

---

[3] A japa mala closely resembles the Christian rosary. For those interested, there is a method of using the fingertips and finger joints to count mantra recitations called *kara mala*. The chanting of mantra by a group with musical accompaniment is called *kirtan*, an increasingly popular yogic technique.

of the word can come into expression, it must be articulated by the throat, mouth, tongue and teeth. It is more accurate to see the practice of japa as placing your body and mind in a dynamic current of energy. By reciting the sounds and words that form the mantra, you entrain this energy and it takes you somewhere.

Japa is often categorized as a concentration practice in which the mantra plays the role of an object of contemplation. While that is certainly true, both the sound of the mantra, and the sentiment with which it is recited, are equally important components. Mantra japa is best understood as an attunement practice meant to harmonize all aspects of your being. The relaxed and rhythmic repetition of the mantra steadies the breath, which slows the heartbeat, and entrains the brain waves. A sense of devotion lowers defenses and brings the emotional faculties online. The cumulative effect synchronizes your system in a way that far exceeds the effects of mental concentration alone.

Every mantra has a literal meaning for the mind to interpret, but its sound, bodily feel, and the breath pattern produced by its repetition are just as important. This combination is how different mantras can be used to create very specialized conditions in the mind and body. Yoga explains this by saying a unique energy is generated by each mantra. Once this is experienced, a person develops great faith in mantra japa. In India, no other practice commands such conviction. It is widely believed that all complaints and sufferings can be remedied by the power embedded in a well-chosen mantra. Everyone knows that even a small obstacle standing in the way of our success can outweigh our good intentions and positive thoughts. A practitioner of japa learns that taking that positive intention and attaching it to a mantra is like firing a shot from a cannon able to destroy such obstacles.

WHAT MANTRA SHOULD I RECITE?

As traditionally taught, a novice yoga student never choses their mantra. Instead, they go to a guru who initiates them into the practice of mantra japa.[4] Whatever mantra they are given is called their guru mantra. It is meant to be recited exactly as instructed, under the auspices of the initiating teacher, who is able to monitor the student's progress and provide continuing guidance. Japa practice always starts with an initial period of intensive recitation called mantra anusthan done to firmly establish the student upon the path of mantra yoga.

> *A student wishing to practice mantra yoga begins with mantra japa. Going to a teacher steeped in mantra shastra (the scriptures that govern mantra yoga), they will be given a mantra and technique that matches their goals and capacity. If japa is to be done for alleviating difficulties or accomplishing any of the first three aims of life, one approach will be taken. If japa is to be done solely in devotion to the Lord and attaining moksha, a different approach will be used. In either case, japa begins with mantra anusthan, an initial practice in which the mantra is repeated many thousands of times.*
>
> *After the number of recitations set by the teacher has been performed, mantra japa consists of performing a prescribed number of malas (yogic rosaries) per day. For example, I ask my students to do a minimum of one mala each morning and evening. Japa should also be practiced in daily life whenever the mind becomes troublesome. This ongoing practice is rightly considered part of mantra anusthan, and it should be carried out without interruption until a student is ready for a next stage of yoga practice. Mantra japa has tremendous power, and practicing in this way will make it available to you.*

DIVINE MANTRAS AND ANAHAT NADA

Swami Kripalu extolled the benefits of reciting what he called *the great mantras of the yoga tradition*, which he believed were received as revelations by its realized sages through the practice of *anahat nada*. Anahat

---

[4] This initiation is called *mantra diksha*. *Anusthan* means "pursuing a goal by persistent action," which in this context means a set and systematic course of mantra repetition.

nada means "the unstruck (not caused by volitional action) sound." This little-known technique and its connection to the yogic mantras is best explained by him:

> *Yoga teaches that all the great mantras (maha mantras) were not composed by human beings. God created and uttered these mantras. How could this be so? When an adept yogi meditates, the nada begins to flow through their subtle body and activates the throat and heart chakras. In this meditative state, all sorts of different sounds begin to flow from their mouth. This experience is called anahat nada or spontaneous sounding. As this sadhana of anahat nada unfolds, the sounds develop into mantras that get repeated again and again to purify, refine, and illuminate the mind of the yogi. In India, these mantras are called "aparushaya," which means "not planned, designed, or created by the mind, but given by grace." This is why these mantras are reverenced and considered of divine origin.*
>
> *None of yoga's great mantras were composed by any particular person. Each of them manifested through anahat nada and evolved into their divine form through the practice of highly realized yogis. In the lineage of gurus to which I belong, there are two such mantras that you should know about. Householders are given the mantra Om Namo Bhagavate Vasudevaya. Renunciate swamis who surrender their life completely to God are given the mantra Om Namah Shivaya.*
>
> *If, out of love for me, you were to compose a new mantra such as Om Namo Kripaluvanada and recite it, you will certainly get the benefit of your focus and faith. But you will not get the full results of mantra japa, because it is not a divine mantra. This is why I instruct students to go to a sadguru (true teacher) to properly receive from them a divine mantra. Then practice it as instructed.*

Repeating a mantra—even a great yogic mantra—alone is not enough. It must be practiced with an understanding of nada that births a mix of confidence and zeal that SK distinguished from "blind faith."

> *The masters of yoga know that mantra recitation must be practiced with conviction. Yet this is not encouraging blind faith—there is*

good reason for it. Our minds are unsteady. Countless thoughts bubble up to the mind's surface only to burst like bubbles in the next moment, which dissipates the mind's energy. Conviction results when we gather this energy by dwelling upon a mantra and its underlying aim. As a result, the mind's energy accumulates and begins to flow in a direct and concentrated way towards accomplishing its purpose. This mental steadiness and energetic power is the ground from which all great and miraculous accomplishments have manifested in the world, and it is cultivated carefully in mantra japa.

BE A DISCERNING STUDENT

A harsh critic could dismiss the whole of mantra yoga as the faith-based use of incantations that delivers its benefits—that is, if there are any—by virtue of the placebo effect. Such opinions are worthy of consideration, but don't end your rational analysis without inquiring into a robust body of research that finds mantra recitation a meditation technique that produces an impressive list of measurable physiological and psychological benefits. Many of those studies were performed in the early days of meditation research and can be found online.

Spiritual teachers can go to the other extreme. The yogic conception of nada is reminiscent of the electromagnetic spectrum that includes radio waves, microwaves, infrared light, visible light, ultraviolet light, X-rays, and gamma rays. A century after its discovery, the electromagnetic spectrum remains a core element of contemporary science that provides an empirical understanding of how the universe operates that undergirds our high-tech world. Some spiritual teachers broaden this scientific model to encompass everything from the densest physical matter to the subtlest spiritual energies. They add to this material spectrum a range of emotional and psychological states that run from those of "low vibration" such as fear, anger, and depression to those of "high vibration" such as love, joy, peace, and bliss.

They may also point to an ultimate reality beyond even the highest vibrational states, describing an Absolute or non-dual ground of being from which all these vibrational manifestations arise. Ideas from the evolving field of quantum physics might be brought in – such as the observer effect, paradox and complementarity, non-locality, particle entanglement, and the role played by "symmetry breaking" in the formation of the early universe—to bolster this view. Mantra meditation might be characterized as a way to replace low vibration thoughts with higher vibration sound formulas. For those adopting this view, the spiritual path becomes a process of learning to resonate at a higher and higher frequencies until the nondual truth of oneness is experienced.

These parallels between science and spirituality are interesting. And admittedly, the model that results from mixing these ideas is on the whole consistent with traditional yoga metaphysics. But it is important for a discerning student to recognize that this expanded version of the electromagnetic spectrum lacks the rigor demanded of hard science. A good bit of what psychologists call intuitive reasoning and several noteworthy leaps of faith are required to bridge these very different models of reality.

Some research studies have compared the meditative use of traditional mantras and other religious dictums with secular words and phrases. Herbert Benson, MD, professor of mind/body medicine at Harvard Medical School, found that using the word "peace" or "one" was equally effective in slowing the heart rate, lowering blood pressure, and eliciting the "relaxation response" he was studying. It should be noted that studies like this typically examine less-experienced meditators seeking to manage stress. While providing important data points, their findings taken alone are insufficient to discredit SK's belief in the power of yogic mantras to foster long-term psychological growth and spiritual awakening. It's possible the colorful origin story he tells of mantra yoga being grounded in the sages' practice of anahat nada only serves to excite faith and encourage focused practice. It's also possible that through trial and error the yogis discovered certain sounds and sonic patterns that stimulate brain centers or produce cognitive effects that we don't yet understand. Considerable research would be required to answer this question definitively.

In my practice, Om has become the cosmic call of the universe and Ram its tuning fork response always reverberating in my heart. Used together or alone, they make it possible to maintain a smooth flow of meditative consciousness with very little mental activity. This suggests to me that other words or sound patterns may have surprising utility.

APPLYING THIS CHAPTER IN PRACTICE

After learning how to do japa, Danna and I completed the 125,000 mantra recitations prescribed for new initiates. Both of us found japa practice calming and centering. It also gave us a vehicle to express our commitment to a path we'd been told would lead us onward to Self-realization. We were still doing two malas per day, as possible given our jobs and other responsibilities, when we moved in as ashram residents.

During our ashram years, neither of us found a name of God or mantra that called to us. Like most residents, we eventually replaced japa with the practice of pranayama and sitting meditation. Our japa story would end there except for an unexpected event that brought home the impact of its practice. It occurred in 2005, a full fifteen years since we had done any japa, and a decade after the ashram scandal brought the whole notion of guru mantra into question.

Late one afternoon, I was driving us home from Kripalu Center after the January board meeting. It was cold and rainy, with temperatures hovering right around freezing. Wending our way down from the high-altitude northern tier of Pennsylvania, we were looking forward to having that mountainous stretch of road in our rear-view mirror. Suddenly and without any warning, we hit a patch of black ice at seventy miles per hour. The car began a slow 360-degree clockwise spin right down the middle of Interstate 81, entirely out of my control. Time slowed as we watched everything rotate around us, knowing that eventually we were going to hit something.

Reflexively, we spoke out in unison a single repetition of the mantra "Om Namo Bhagavate Vasudevaya." In the second or two it took to slowly say those words, we came fully present to the reality of what was happening, and placed our lives in God's hands. Sliding into the highway median, time speeded back up as the car roughly ploughed to a stop. It took a few minutes to determine that neither of us was hurt, thanks to all the snow that had cushioned the impact. Gathering our wits, I did a little shoveling and was able to maneuver the car safely back on the road without anyone's assistance. I was hoping to limp to the next exit and find a repair shop, but the car accelerated easily and seemed no worse for its careening.

We'd planned on getting home that night, but further driving was out of the question. Still inwardly shaking, we stopped at a hotel north of Harrisburg. To have escaped unscathed from this life-threatening experience felt miraculous. Clasping each other as if to make sure that both of us were still in one piece, we struggled to understand where the mantra had come from. Neither of us had any sense of starting it. To this day, we have no explanation except the obvious. In a moment of free fall, it surfaced from the depths of our psyches to give us something positive to voice and hold onto.

Sharing this personal anecdote turns my mind to the much more significant story of Mahatma Gandhi, whose masterful leadership of the Indian independence movement is often cited to confirm his greatness as a karma yogi. Yet his spiritual greatness might be equally evident in his mantra yoga and death. Weak from fasting to protest the interfaith religious violence that had broken out in the run up to Independence Day, the seventy-eight-year-old Gandhi was on his way to a prayer meeting when a man emerged from the admiring crowd. After bowing, the man shot him three times at point-blank range in the stomach and chest. Gandhi raised his hands in front of his face in prayer positioning, saluting his assassin. Slumping to the ground, the last words from his lips were his lifelong mantra: "Ram, Ram."

Readers wanting to apply the content of this chapter in practice are likely to run into an immediate hurdle. I am not aware of any teachers in SK's lineage who are initiating and guiding students in mantra japa. Despite his emphasis on finding a qualified teacher, SK always maintained that a sincere seeker could obtain what he called "initiation from a distance" as explained below. Our exploration of mantra yoga practice continues in the next chapter.

A seeker cannot expect to begin mantra yoga without securing a benediction to embark upon its path. Mantra diksha (initiation) is that through which one formally attains this permission to practice. If a seeker cannot visit an able guru in person, but studies well their writings, and sincerely practices their teachings as instructed therein, and has great faith, they will be able to obtain initiation from a distance. Another avenue to this initiation is the grace of God, and anyone who chants the name of the Lord with love will receive this grace automatically. But seekers should realize that the true path of yoga is one of overcoming obstacles. Just as patients should consult a physician, and students a professor, a yogic aspirant should find a way to consult with an adept yoga master to ensure their proper practice and progress.

CHAPTER 19
MANTRA YOGA IN PRACTICE

Mantra yoga is a path well-suited to those living active lives. Yet its basis is the sadhana of anahat nada done by reclusive yogis, which produces the sound formulas that when repeated by anyone under proper conditions bring about extraordinary results. In truth, the practitioners of these paths evolve together.

Mantra japa and mantra yoga are not synonyms. Mantra yoga is a multi-stage path of yoga complete unto itself. Mantra japa as presented in the last chapter is one of its preliminary techniques. After learning and mastering this basic technique, Swami Kripalu taught that a deepening mantra yoga practice generally takes one of three forms.

In the first, the practice of japa continues in a manner designed to cultivate states of divine contact and communion that lead devotees toward God-realization. In the second, the practice of japa is replaced with an altogether different technique, mantra meditation, done by those of a contemplative bent to render the mind thoughtless, after which more advanced meditation techniques like inner sound meditation are employed. The third form of mantra yoga practice cannot be volitionally adopted; it has to occur naturally. This is the phenomenon of spontaneous sounding or anahat nada that was touched upon in the last chapter and is referenced in the above epigraph. This chapter addresses each of these mantra yoga sub-paths.

At first, a yogic aspirant does mantra japa to escape the menace of the thinking mind. Here a question arises: Why this aversion towards the mind and thoughts? We all know that extraneous thoughts steal away our mental peace. But it may not be known that as soon as thoughts cease, the activity of the mind also ceases, and all awareness of the physical self disappears. When this occurs, a faith-oriented practitioner of japa who utters mantra as God's name will feel as if they have been taken to the kingdom of heaven. A truth-seeking practitioner of japa who gives primary importance to meditation will experience this fixity of mind (dharana) as a doorway into the formless realms of dhyana and samadhi. After this occurrence, it does not matter whether one continues to perform the japa of God's name and have divine experiences, or begins the practice of yogic meditation. Either path will ultimately lead to the mind's dissolution into the source of its origin. A third category of yogic aspirant experiences mantra occurring entirely of its own accord. This spontaneous sounding (anahat nada) results when an aspirant's life energy awakens and causes countless sounds to issue forth directly from the energy centers (chakras). While taking different pathways, all of these aspirants have found a known way to make the journey of yoga.

MANTRA JAPA FOR DIVINE CONTACT AND COMMUNION

As previously noted, the majority of SK's students were devotees who practiced mantra yoga as an extension of their Hindu religious faith. For these students, a modified version of mantra japa remained core to their spiritual life. Before examining the advanced expression of the basic japa technique, an upfront caveat is warranted. SK saw this version of mantra japa as only suited to his *faithful students*, meaning theists. Without a devotional orientation, he felt its practice would neither make sense nor call forth the zeal required for its effectiveness:

Atheists and intellectuals are only being consistent when they criticize mantra chanting as foolish. If there is no Supreme Being, how could reciting the Divine name have any effect? I allow such intellectuals their ideas, while guiding faithful students along the path of master yogis who realized the highest through mantra japa. Everyone acknowledges the names of great people and well-known places. A mere mention is enough to bring their object to mind. Surely then, the countless names of God are at least of equal import. The more a japa yogi becomes intimate with their chosen name and form (ishta devata), the more they appreciate its power to bring the Lord present. A person calling on the telephone of mantra gets answered right away because it is directed to a name and number given us by God himself (through anahat nada). In this entire world, there is no technique that has produced as many miracles as repeating the names of the divine. In fact, the biggest of all miracles (God realization) is hidden in every such name and obtainable by reciting it in mantra japa or chanting it in kirtan (the musical praising of the Lord).

A pillar of the Hindu faith is espoused in the two-word term *ishta devata*, which means "cherished deity." It's widely known that Indian religion includes an exotic array of gods and goddesses. It's less understood that a devout Hindu is expected to choose a particular form of God for whom they feel the greatest affinity. This ishta devata becomes the primary object of their devotion and worship. In order to engage in depth mantra japa, a specific name and form must be selected. In fact, the selection of an ishta devata is meant to reflect a lifelong religious choice. At times, a yogic aspirant might recite the name or mantra of a god or goddess whose distinctive attributes can help them overcome a specific problem or satisfy a particular desire, in much the same way that a Catholic Christian might pray to a patron saint, but that orientation is short-term and more aligned with the basic japa technique described in the prior chapter.

SK established the philosophical basis for this depth practice in an instructional pamphlet given to everyone who came to him for mantra initiation. Its title reflects the goal of advanced japa practice: *Marga Darshan*, which means The Way to Divine Presence:

With affection and concern for my spiritual well-being, my guru taught me the truth of monotheism (ekeshvaravad). God is One, but human beings offer their worship in different ways. Accordingly,

I honor the innumerable names and forms of the Infinite and Almighty. Just by uttering any of these names with total love and devotion, an individual's sins and deficiencies can be brought to an end and spiritual salvation gained. To ensure your well-being, I impart this same teaching to you. Consider each of the many divine names as sacred and all the many forms of God as worthy of worship. Never demean any of these names or forms. Never criticize or hate anyone belonging to a different sect or faith. Never denounce their sacred scriptures or express displeasure at their holy saints. Renounce your ignorance and accept that all these faiths and sects eventually merge into the holy feet of the One Great God. Whatever form of God you like most, that calls forth your love, and to which you feel attuned, worship It (your ishta devata) in this spirit.

Make no mistake, this form of mantra japa is a yogic rite performed to invoke what SK sometimes called the Supreme Spirit (Paramatman) by reciting the name and envisioning the form of a specific god or goddess.[1] Practicing this form of japa wholeheartedly requires the faith born of a theistic view, a notion that he reinforces again and again.

Each mantra is linked with a particular god or goddess. Hence, in order to have the darshan (audience) of that deity, one worships It through the medium of mantra japa. Mantras chanted for this purpose are considered the subtle body of the deity expressing its distinctive consciousness and energy. But mouthing the mantra is

---

[1] All the major faiths have some form of spiritual practice in which a short prayer or name of the divine is repeated intently or incessantly to keep the mind focused on God. Christians have used the prayer "Lord Jesus Christ, have mercy upon me," as presented in the classic nineteenth-century text, *The Way of a Pilgrim*. Muslims repeat the name of Allah in a practice called dhikr which means "to remember." Some Sufi orders sharply accent the first syllable, which activates the in-breath. Others extend the sounding of its second syllable as long as the breath allows, prolonging the outbreath. Either way converts the Islamic name of God into the equivalent of a yogic mantra. While non-theistic, Buddhists are no exception. Tibetan Buddhism has a rich lexicon of mantras including Om Mani Padme Hum, which means "Om, behold/hail the jewel in the lotus" and is recited to invoke Avalokitesvara, the Buddha of Compassion. Members of the Japanese sect of Nichiren Buddhism recite the phrase "Nam Myoho Renge Kyo," which literally means "I take refuge in the Lotus of the Wonderful Law," to erase individual karma and awaken the Buddha nature of all beings. Many more examples could be given.

not enough. The cold water in a steam engine produces no result. Only when a fire is kindled and the water is brought to a boil does the engine come to life. Similarly, it is only when mantra chanting and devotion are brought together that the power inherent in the mantra gets unlocked. Millions of devoted men and women have crossed the ocean of frustration and realized new lives by having the darshan of their chosen form of the Lord. This is a fundamental truth of bhakti yoga.

Swami Kripalu considered this form of mantra yoga well-suited to householders because it could be sustained with a modest daily practice. The kind of intensive practice required for breakthroughs and quantum leaps could be done periodically away from home in a retreat setting, after which daily japa practice would resume its role as an anchor in their spiritual life. SK's guidance on "How to Do a Mantra Japa Retreat" can be found in Appendix 3.

A devotee uses the practice of japa to forge an intimate relationship with their ishta devata. Repeating the name of their beloved Lord, their only desire is to bask in the divine presence. There is little talk on this subpath of divine union or non-duality, the explicit goal of many more-meditative yoga schools. Yet bhakti yoga recognizes that God's presence is intoxicating. It often causes a devotee to lose their self-sense and merge with the deity in moments that transcend words or thoughts. While a japa practitioner seeks nothing beyond divine communion, grace may carry them beyond the conventional subject/object distinctions underlying worship and mantra recitation. This is bhakti yoga's approach to God-realization, and its efficacy is why SK considered mantra japa a complete yogic path.

MANTRA MEDITATION

Like japa, mantra meditation makes use of a sacred sound formula. But the similarities end there. Mantra meditation is not an extension of japa—it is a new and altogether different technique whose purpose is to render the mind thoughtless. The distinction between these two practices must be held in mind to grasp the purpose of mantra meditation and understand the two stages through which it is practiced.

To begin mantra sadhana, assume a posture in which you can sit comfortably. Remain quiet for a few moments to allow the mind to settle. Then inwardly say a prayer or affirmation of your choice, expressing your devotion and inclining the mind toward introversion. If you wish to give importance to the recitation of a mantra including God's name, consider meditation to be subsidiary and begin your japa. If you wish to give importance to meditation, attend to the breath and use a mantra such as Soham, Rama, or Om to absorb the attention in the flow of inhalations and exhalations. This entry into meditation is well known, and any mantra that eases the breath may be used. Mantra yoga does not instruct a seeker to either praise God in form (Saguna Brahman) by doing japa or silently meditate on the formless Absolute (Nirguna Brahman). Choose either way according to your liking.

The mantras traditionally used in japa are relatively long—ranging between five and thirty-two syllables. For example, "Om Namah Shivaya" as pronounced is a crisp five syllables. "Om Namo Bhagavata Vasudevaya" has twelve; the Gayatri Mantra has twenty-four; and the Mahamantra, made famous by the Hare Krishnas, has thirty-two. They often begin with the seed syllable Om and then venerate a particular deity who is succinctly referenced, usually by name. By comparison, the mantras used in mantra meditation are short, often two syllables that flow nicely with the breath. In advanced practice, the mantra may be shortened to a single one-syllable word. Western studies suggest the word "peace" works well as a meditation mantra.

In the first stage of practice, the mantra is recited with the natural flow of breath. For example, a practitioner may inwardly say the word "peace" each time the breath flows in, and say the word "peace" again as the breath flows out. This stage of practice is called breath-assisted repetition. If done with a relaxed focus, it curbs extraneous thoughts and causes the thought stream passing through the mind to gradually slow down. If that focus is sustained over time, the recitation of the single word "peace" in rhythm with the breath will winnow all other thoughts from the mind. That's the purpose of breath-assisted repetition. Everyone sits down to meditate with a head full of thoughts. This technique is meant to quickly bring a practitioner to a mental state of one-pointedness in which the idea and feeling of peace permeate the body-mind. For someone skilled in breath-assisted repetition, the need to recite the mantra in rhythm with the breath will soon give way to a subtler sense of hearing the mantra moving with the breath, as if it were being spoken by a third-party in the background. The mental passivity inherent in simply listening to the sound of the mantra—versus having to generate and give voice to it—allows the mind to grow very quiet.

The second stage of mantra meditation is called "Repetition Without Support." A practitioner lets go of any link between the breath and the recitation of the mantra. At first, this shift in technique may occur as abrupt and mentally disruptive. If so, the word "peace" may need to be repeated several times in succession to return to the state of one-pointedness. But once this bridge has been crossed, it becomes possible to rest for moments in a more spacious state that SK called *thoughtlessness*, which just as aptly could be called "presence."

At first, these moments are likely to be brief, but the technique of mantra yoga provides a tool to return again and again to the thoughtless state. Whenever the thinking mind comes back in and a practitioner finds themselves distracted or lost in story, they break the flow of thought by mentally saying "peace." This is done gently so as to not further activate the mind. Just reintroducing the notion of the word, without having to recite or hear it, is often sufficient. Once again, rest in the thoughtless state.

> *As soon as a meditator closes their eyes, they discover a large congregation of competing thoughts gathered in their mind. Unless a technique is known, their effort to obtain peace will be wasted. Two different keys unlock the technique of mantra meditation. First, only desired thoughts (those related to the mantra) are allowed to remain in the mind—others are simply ignored. Next, the mantra is used to ease the breath and curb (slow down) the pace of remaining thoughts. With this technique alone, it is possible to experience a single-mindedness that ends in thoughtlessness. The thoughtless state is also experienced in deep sleep, where it is always restorative, but thoughtlessness by itself is not illuminating. To whatever extent you can merge your thoughtless mind into beyond-mind awareness,*

to that extent your success in meditation can be measured. After the mind has been thus introverted and rendered thoughtless in the meditation room, its extroverted nature of continuous thinking will reassert itself outside the meditation room. A meditator should expect that back and forth to continue until the mind has truly been transcended in superconscious samadhi.

In this second stage of mantra meditation practice, it's fine for periods of time to pass in which the practitioner entirely forgets they are repeating the word "peace." The objective is not to repeat or even remember the word, but to rest in moments of inner peace and thought-free awareness. During these moments of mental stillness, mantra yoga teaches that you are being informed by the cosmic mind and its profound ordering intelligence.

When a child is born in your home, what name to call it is up to you. It's the same when the idea of God is born in your mind. When you are choosing among all the divine names, remember one thing said by all the sages. Ram and Om are the best names upon which to meditate. Ram will purify the lower centers, open the heart, and call the mind away from the world of form. Om will bring you into oneness with the formless God. First use the word Ram, either in chanting or meditation, until the mind is engrossed and everything else is forgotten. Then allow your mind and Om to merge together.

Despite his theistic disposition, SK was quick to say to say that all these principles of mantra yoga can be applied to a non-theistic form of breath-based meditation able to deliver the same results:

A silent form of breath meditation may also be practiced in which the sadhak (practitioner) closely observes his breath. This is the meditation taught in Buddhist religion, which can be practiced whether or not you accept the idea of God or an Absolute level of existence. Bring awareness to the movement of the breath. Whenever the attention wanders, a patient effort should be made to reestablish concentration on the breath. In this way, the constant movement of the mind and its flow of one distracting thought after another can be gradually curbed. Yoga calls this breath meditation ajapa japa (japa without a mantra) and it also opens into the realm of thoughtless meditation.

For more instructions on how to practice Mantra Meditation, see Appendix 3.

GOING FURTHER ON THE PATH OF MANTRA MEDITATION

Mantra meditation uses mantra recitation as a tool to coalesce the mind around a single thought. Then the tool of mantra is set aside to rest in the thoughtless state. SK considered the ability to access this state—if only for brief moments—a threshold skill anyone wanting to practice depth yogic meditation must develop. Once the process of crossing the bridge to thoughtlessness has grown familiar, some other technique of what he called *formless meditation* should be engaged that is aimed directly at samadhi and Self-realization. Out of many possible such techniques, two are so closely associated with mantra yoga that they deserve mention here. The first is inner sound meditation. The second is anahat nada.

INNER SOUND MEDITATION

Poised in the thoughtless state, an alert meditator may begin to notice a world of inner sounds. At first, the sounds heard may be quite ordinary. The sound of breath moving in and out of the lungs. The beat of the heart. Blood circulating through various parts of the body. But as the mind grows increasingly quiet, a progression of subtler sounds may begin to emerge from the background. If that occurs, meditation can become a process of listening and attuning to these inner sounds.

It's important to acknowledge that most meditators never encounter this inner soundscape. Yet for those who do, it grants an opportunity to explore the phenomenon of nada firsthand. Practitioners often describe this process as tuning into an auditory frequency that has always been there, except their mind was too busy to notice it. The true goal of this practice is not so much to hear these inner sounds, but to sink into the silence and mental stillness that intent listening generates.

Yoga teaches that as these inner sounds grow increasingly subtle, you are led into a progression of deeper mind states. Step by step, your awareness is being naturally guided back to nada's point of origin: the silent source from which subtle sound (nada), spiritual light (jyoti), and life force (prana) emanate. There are many approaches to inner sound meditation but one keystone idea unites them. The sounds will grow increasingly subtle until one is heard that is noticeably different because of its steadiness. As that steady sound is meditated upon, it will gradually evolve into an expression of the Om mantra. When the inner sound stabilizes, a meditator is guided to merge their attention into it to transcend all mental activity. SK reinforces this theme and touches on many other facets of the practice in this instructive excerpt:

> *The Nada Bindu Upanishad says, "A yogi seated in meditation posture should listen with the right ear to the unstruck inner sound." The instructions on how to do this nada meditation are not complicated. Whatever the yogi finds within their range of hearing in the form of nada (inner sound that is spontaneously occurring), intently meditate upon that as a subtle expression of the formless God.*
>
> *There are innumerable inner sounds, which may be divided into the three classes, subtle, subtler, and subtlest. Enchanted by these sounds, the mental faculty effortlessly becomes one-pointed and serene. Listening to ever subtler sounds, the mind is led toward samadhi. In the beginning, an aspirant might hear the sound of the ocean, a cascading waterfall, the rumble of a thunderhead, or a kettledrum. After that, drums of all kinds, gongs and tinkling bells, conchs and horns, all sorts or stringed instruments, flutes and high-pitched sounds resembling the buzzing of insects, and celestial music or singing. Some of these sounds may seem to be situated at specific places in the body.*
>
> *Reading this description, a student might ask: Inside the human body or brain is there a storehouse of instruments similar to what might be found in the music department of a college? That*

might be followed by another question. How are these sounds generated? I have found it unproductive to spend much time searching for answers to questions such as this, as yet science has no response. All that can be truly said is that yogis from ancient times to now do in fact hear these sounds.

In this method, the mental faculty should be allowed to stroll up and down the scales of these sounds, lost in delight and forgetting the outside world. It should not be made to go anywhere particular, as that sound in which the mind naturally becomes engrossed is the best one for creating absorption. Listening to it will result in the mind becoming stable. Compared to the pranav mantra (Om), all these other sounds are not very important. Om is expressive of the Highest Absolute, and it alone carries the mind into divine absorption (samadhi).

For a set of simple instructions on how to practice Inner Sound Meditation, see Appendix 3.

SPONTANEOUS SOUNDING OR ANAHAT NADA

Focused mantra or inner sound meditation—or any other yogic practice done intensively—can galvanize an energy awakening that sometimes shifts, and other times catapults, a practitioner into the experience of anahat nada or "spontaneous sounding," which is the most-advanced technique of mantra yoga. This is the path that presented itself to SK, which leads to a dynamic form of meditation totally unlike inner sound meditation.[2] Instead of reciting a traditional mantra given by an outside authority, the practitioner utters only those sounds and words arising from their direct energetic connection to Spirit.

When a highly developed seeker meditates and causes the throat chakra to activate, all sorts of sounds begin to flow spontaneously out the mouth. Some yell, others chant known mantras, some repeat prayers in languages unknown to them, still other sing and dance.

[2] SK did not access the thoughtless state through mantra meditation, but via the intensive practice of anuloma viloma pranayama, which led to his energy awakening and practice of anahat nada. For more, see chapter 4 of *Dharma Then Moksha*.

> *All these different expressions of nada manifest automatically without any apparent cause. A seeker cannot continue this meditation without gaining the ability to surrender completely to the cosmic energy that is propelling these actions. All of these manifestations are to be welcomed, with none resisted or stopped. The scriptures say that such a seeker will eventually utter the pranav mantra (Om) and complete the path of yoga. But making little headway, they soon realize that years of solitary sadhana stand between them and this goal. It is at this point that the inadequacy of self-guided efforts is accepted, and the necessity of obtaining the guidance of an experienced yogi guru is understood.*

It is misguided to think that instruction can be given on the practice of anahat nada, which is not a yogic technique but rather a yogic experience. But SK did provide instruction on how to chant Om in a way that could lead into the experience of anahat nada—see page Appendix 3. He also told the story of a novice student who quickly progressed to the practice of Anahat Nada—see Appendix 2.

BE A DISCERNING STUDENT

Swami Kripalu practiced mantra japa religiously from childhood until age thirty-eight, when he began intensive pranayama. Pranayama generated a hybrid state of high energy and thoughtlessness, the combination of which thrust him on the path of anahat nada. Active sounding carried him into states of depth meditation in which he heard the inner sounds. Having walked this particular pathway, his teachings on mantra meditation are somewhat limited.

After leaving the ashram, I wanted to know more and branched out to study TM—Transcendental Meditation—as taught by Maharishi Mahesh Yogi, and Centering Prayer as taught by Father Thomas Keating, OCSO. As my practice of mantra meditation deepened, I became interested in inner sound meditation as presented in the Kriya Yoga tradition of Paramahansa Yogananda, including the teachings of his disciple, Roy Eugene Davis. When an area of interest captures your attention, I encourage you to broaden your horizons in similar ways. I've distilled what I learned into the two instructional handouts in Appendix 3.

SK's teaching that mantra meditation should eventually be followed by additional techniques of *formless meditation* because *thoughtlessness by itself is not illuminating* is unconventional. Adept mantra meditators are generally guided to set the mantra aside and rest in pure consciousness, an approach deemed sufficient for Self-realization. I found this experience profound—and often light-filled—but returning there again and again my meditation practice eventually stagnated. That led me to continue to explore other techniques, the most notable of which for me has been Self-inquiry. Through ongoing practice, I've come to agree with the point SK was making, which I would express a little differently: thoughtlessness by itself is not enlightening.

APPLYING THIS CHAPTER IN PRACTICE

I've only met one adept practitioner of inner sound meditation, but the encounter was edifying enough to recount here. Danna and I were at Spirit Rock Meditation Center teaching yoga classes for participants in a Vipassana meditation retreat. We quickly became friends with Robert Hall, a retired psychiatrist and one of Spirit Rock's senior teachers. Every day at lunchtime, the three of us would sit together in the faculty yurt and eagerly converse.

One afternoon, I happened to express my interest in inner sound meditation and Robert's eyebrows shot up. Within moments, he was telling me how he and his ex-wife had been initiated into the practice by a yogic guru in the 1970s. Both of them were so taken by the power of this technique that they converted the master bedroom closet of their San Francisco home into a sound-proofed meditation room, as external silence was an important element in the approach in which they were being schooled. As a psychiatrist and spiritual teacher, Robert believed in the value of awareness-based Vipassana meditation. But eventually he found his progress petering out and worse yet his desire to practice drying up. At that point, he returned to listening to the rich soundscape of inner sounds with renewed enthusiasm. All the time we had been sitting in the dharma hall together, it was not Vipassana but inner sound meditation that Robert was doing, a practice he deemed a perfect match for the silent environment that Buddhist retreat centers like Spirit Rock offer.

Robert was a man of real stature, highly regarded by his Vipassana colleagues, to the extent that Danna and I were floored by this private revelation. Setting that aside, I listened closely to the practical guidance he offered me, which differed markedly from the way Swami Kripalu spoke of the practice. This discrepancy alerted me to the existence of two alternate approaches to hearing these inner sounds. In the first, a novice practitioner strives to discern these subtle sounds by practicing in pin drop silence. Meditation is done in the wee hours of the morning when noise is at a minimum. Yogic mudras (bodily positions) may be assumed that close the ears with the palms or thumbs, or a T-shaped "meditation crutch" may be used to block the ears without straining the arms. SK's teachings reflect an entirely different approach in which the life energy (prana) is raised—usually through a combination of spartan diet, celibacy, rigorous hatha yoga, and intensive pranayama—to the point where these inner sounds become audible without any external supports. Both of these approaches are yogically advanced and meant to be adopted by meditators who have mastered basic techniques like japa and mantra meditation. Each is meant to give rise to the Om mantra and ultimately dissolve the mind into the silence underlying all sound.

It's two decades since I had the good fortune to befriend Robert Hall. Periods of inner sounding come and go in my meditation life, and seem more sidelight than focal point. Quite often, I awake to these sounds naturally accompanying my movement out of sleep. At times while meditating, I will notice a faint and often high-pitched sound that when attended to grows discernable then rich. At its best, my experience is a little like being outside on a summer night, when the crickets, cicadas, katydids, and tree frogs all contribute to a chorus that captures and carries away the attention. Often those experiences end with a state I'd describe as listening to the silence itself.

We are all trying to navigate the turbulent waters of life. Not everyone can do hatha yoga or meditation. But anyone can choose a mantra and repeat it to incline their mind in a positive direction. It may be just be the syllable Ram, but consider it your sacred word and return to it continually. Much like a person in the oceans who holds fast to a piece of wood, a yogi who makes of their mantra a raft need not fear whirlpools or drowning.

CHAPTER 20
SKILLFULNESS IN ACTION

> *If someone in ancient India said the word yoga, it meant karma yoga unless a different meaning was specified. That's how central the path of action was to the rishis and sages. Today yoga schools are numerous but few make mention of karma yoga. Yet each of them must give importance to skillful action as without it success in any domain of life is not possible.*

Danna and I spent the summer after my graduation from law school living at Kripalu Center as volunteers in the Karma Yoga Training Program. Arriving there, we joined an eclectic group of fifty individuals from all over North America and Europe. In return for the ability to take part in the yoga classes and spiritual life of the ashram, we were willing to work nine hours each day, six-and-a-half days a week. Despite the name of the program in which we had enrolled, we saw it as work-exchange. None of us had signed up to learn the "yoga of action."

Danna was assigned to veggie prep with a dozen other "sisters" who did the staggering amount of knife work necessary to feed the 300-person vegetarian community. I was put on dish crew, a parallel team of "brothers" who washed the mountain of plates, bowls, utensils, cups, and trays that piled up after each meal in what everyone called the dining chapel. The program had a modular curriculum that included sessions on many facets of yogic living, but its overarching purpose was to teach us how to work mindfully in a relaxed and efficient manner, discharging our duties with an attitude of selfless service to the community. Morale among the volunteers was high, and it was inspiring to see everyone taking pride in their work and doing it with excellence.

> *The Bhagavad Gita defines karma yoga as skillfulness in action, but to acquire this capacity you need a discipline and setting in which to practice it. Service is such an effective discipline for developing the artfulness in action signified by the term karma yoga that it surpasses any other instrument that may be employed. While an ashram setting is the optimal training ground, the tool of service can be usefully applied anywhere.*

We arrived as a committed couple. We'd lived together for the previous school year and were formally engaged to be married. But to participate in the program, we had to agree to live separately on the same terms as the other single volunteers. Socializing or even talking with members of the opposite sex was strictly off limits. As the program neared its completion, we got permission to meet privately and compare notes. Each of us had learned a lot from our solo experience, but neither of us wanted to stay on as ashram residents, which would have meant four more years of living singly before we could enter the relationships program. So we left Kripalu Center intent on applying everything we'd learned at home in our married life and also in our work settings.

One big takeaway from our volunteer experience was learning that karma yoga was not about performing any special actions. It was the discipline of staying present to what was happening in the moment, then bringing consciousness and caring to bear upon each and every action performed throughout the day. Yet I knew from reading the Bhagavad Gita that there was more to know, which led me to delve into Swami Kripalu's teachings. That's where I learned that karma yoga is meant to progress through its own series of stages that start where character building leaves off.

In character building, you dynamically pursue your purpose and aims in life while acting in an honest, straightforward, and increasingly principled manner. Karma yoga teaches you how to continue this growth by adopting an attitude of *seva*, a common word in the ashram lexicon that means *service*.

SK ON SEVA

Seva is the first step on a staircase called "karma yoga" by which one can walk all the way to the kingdom of heaven. Climbing it is a challenging task, as each step unfolds more and more of a person's divinity. Before undertaking the ascent of this staircase, one must possess a love for good character, as without this valuing of virtue, the practice of karma yoga cannot succeed.

"Seva" means "service" but that is only its ordinary definition. You can understand its deeper meaning by examining the mechanism of your own body, which contains many organs. Although the roles and functional interests of the organs are distinct, there is no disharmony among them. Instead, there is unity of purpose in the midst of diverse activity. By being entirely devoted to its function, each organ uplifts the health of all the others. In the same way, you can dedicate yourself to your particular purpose and duties in life while adopting an attitude of service to the whole.

Setting aside your wants to serve the collective good may sound like sacrifice. Yet there is no more profitable transaction than seva. In truth, seva is a peculiar form of selfishness, as those who live only for themselves inevitably meet with unhappiness, while serving others is the infallible way to gain happiness. Charitable actions performed with a self-serving motive and carried out in a conspicuous manner are registered in society's logbook. But seva rendered inconspicuously is noted in God's logbook. As possible, service should be done in an unpretentious manner, as this is how one's underlying humility comes forth. The impetus for seva arises not only from the purity of the heart and mind but also from the depth of the soul. The soul's activation marks the end of the initial stage of seva, after which the higher stages of karma yoga can unfold.

A person practicing seva ceases to play the game of life solely for themselves. Psychologically speaking, this is no small matter. SK recognized that the transition from character building to karma yoga must be a gradual one. I was inspired by the idealistic instruction given in the Bhagavad Gita: "Let thy aim be the good of all and carry on thy tasks in life." (3:20.) But I also took heed of SK's advice to proceed along this *path of consecrated action* gradually.

Karma Yoga is the basis of all yoga. To master any of its pathways, a student must practice this yoga of action. But first it may be necessary to dispel an erroneous notion. The Gita says a karma yogi should act without any attachment to the fruit of his actions. While this is true, a beginning student must perform action with some expectation of results. We all try to meet our needs by acting in ways informed by our previous efforts in life. My guru taught me that you must start your karma yoga practice motivated by desire (satkam), as only after a practice has matured will actions become desireless (nishkam).

A person who works only for wages is correctly categorized as a laborer and not a karma yogi. But a person who works to meet the needs of himself and his family, attentively doing his work with devotion in the spirit of karma yoga, belongs to a second category. A person able to perform desireless actions as a holy sacrifice for the good of all beings without any attachment to results belongs to a third category.

A yogi comes into this third category of practice only at the very end of the path. Long before this, each of us must be willing to commence our practice of yogic action, accepting in advance wherever it might lead us. This is the non-attachment required to start upon the path of consecrated action, which must then be walked with faith and firm determination.

Before I could undertake the practice of non-attachment, I had to understand exactly what this word was meant to convey. To do that, I turned to a verse of the Bhagavad Gita that was among SK's favorites: "Set thy heart upon thy work, but never on its rewards. Your right is to action alone, and never to its fruits. Overcome inertia and energetically perform your duties in peace, abandoning any attachment to their success or failure. This evenness of mind is yoga." (2:47-48)

It would be nice to report that my progress along the path of karma yoga was immediate and swift, but I actually found this instruction impossible to implement. All I could genuinely do was carry on in my practice of service, which was well suited to the legal aid work in which I was engaged. My exploration of non-attachment only began five years later when Danna and I returned to ashram residency. But that intervening time was important for it enabled me to learn the ropes of lawyering and become comfortable in my role as a client advocate.

While serving as Kripalu Center's lawyer, I worked hand-in-glove with the management team and board, where important decisions were made through a group process. All sorts of factors were at play beyond my legal opinion, so it made sense to set my preferences aside and allow for co-creative outcomes to take shape. As I grew acquainted with being "out of control," I discovered it was possible to stop strategizing about how to produce any particular result and tune into my sense of rightness in the moment. This was a new and different practice, and through it I became more intuitively guided in my speech and actions. Practicing non-attachment did not liberate me from having to think cogently, which in my role as a lawyer was essential. But much of the time I could set aside worry, and all the obsessive patterns that accompanied it, to focus on the issues at hand. This approach worked. As I grew to trust it, my actions—just as SK predicted—became more proficient:

For a yogi able to abandon attachment, karma yoga ceases to be an ordinary path. It becomes an extraordinary path upon which one learns to act intuitively from a direct connection to reality. Those who follow this path find the knowledge of how to act arising spontaneously and they are progressively relieved of a sense of doership. Ceaselessly they continue to act, yet they no longer feel they are the doers of those actions. Witnessing how all these actions are automatically generated, they consider themselves to be only an instrument, an object used by the Divine will. Their only desire becomes to serve this Divine will with a consecrated intellect. But the liberation-seeking karma yogi must abandon even this wish as yet another attachment. However, it is not correct to treat this final desire as an ordinary desire, as that will prevent emancipation. This final wish is different because it is merely the ash remaining from the annihilation of all other desires. As such, it is easily swept away by the breeze of grace.

As the above teaching makes clear, coupling the discipline of karma yoga with non-attachment is a potent and potentially liberating practice. The Bhagavad Gita points out the final step on the path of karma yoga in a single verse: "Let the wise man work selflessly for the good of all the world." (3:25) Thankfully, SK commented on what this means:

The service of a student and the service of a siddha (great master) are not the same. Students aspire to serve with a selfless attitude. To whatever extent they purify their intention, their service prepares them for the unfolding of the higher mind. Depending on their disposition and circumstances in life, a student may or may not engage in public service. But whenever this higher mind expresses through a master, it always takes the form of service to the people.

History shows that every great master has done this service to society. Why is this so? Only one who has more capacity can serve. The rich can serve the poor; the learned can serve the uneducated; the healthy can serve the unhealthy. A master realizes that service can't be rendered to God, who possesses all. Nor can service be rendered to their guru, who has already realized the truth and may have left this world. So a great master serves the people, seeing them as an expression of the Supreme itself.

BE A DISCERNING STUDENT

Yoga came to America at the close of the nineteenth century, and the yoga movement has been growing in size and sophistication ever since. Generally speaking, its early leaders and teachers had their hands full popularizing the practice of physical yoga and educating the public on the benefits of meditation. During this phase of yoga's development, yoga enthusiasts tended to see themselves as creating an alternative community distinct from mainstream culture. Perhaps as a result, many yogis were not socially or politically active. Their practice of karma yoga was expressed through serving their guru (teacher) and insular yoga ashram (center), sangha (community), or kula (family or tribe).

Today, the yoga movement has come of age. Along with that, the tenor of the times has shifted. Now many of the best-known yogis are outspoken activists seeking to foster social justice, remedy climate change, and otherwise raise the mainstream consciousness. Their actions mesh with the legacy of many noteworthy yogic saints, including SK, who spent many years serving and uplifting society.

In ancient times, temples were the fountains from which yogic principles flowed into Indian culture. It was these temples, and the holy saints who established them, that gave birth to innumerable selfless works and many institutions that even now continue to operate. It is my hope that today's spiritual centers will spread yoga all over the world. To do so, they must become centers of service established by saintly well-wishers of society and watchful leaders ever thinking about the welfare, needs, and grievances of the people. True yoga always acts to uplift the individual, family, and society. That's why the best way to bring yoga to the world is to simultaneously practice yoga, operate spiritual centers, and engage in social action.

While the maturation of the yoga movement should be celebrated, any tendency to see karma yoga as synonymous with social activism should be questioned and considered too narrow in accord with its broader definition "skillfulness in action" as presented above. Remember, karma yoga is not about taking any particular kind of actions. It is the discipline of staying present to life and bringing awakened consciousness and caring to bear upon each and every action performed throughout the day.

APPLYING THIS CHAPTER IN PRACTICE

As SK pointed out, genuine seva is usually the result of a lengthy developmental process. This is evident in the lives of many laudable civic leaders and philanthropists, who spend years establishing themselves in successful careers before using their position to help others by serving on nonprofit boards and financially supporting beneficial causes. Alongside performing good deeds, the acts of a true karma yogi are undergirded by a consciousness identified with all of existence. Feeling connected to the whole of society, the impetus to serve arises from a natural inclination to be of benefit, especially to those less fortunate.

Aspiring students are directed to the Bhagavad Gita, whose potent teachings have stood the test of time. While continuing your studies there, avoid the pitfall of thinking you can implement all its advice at once. While you don't have to be an activist to put the principles of karma yoga into action, you do need a discipline to bring them to life.

Start where you are by seeing everything you are already doing from the perspective of service, and let your path unfold from there.

SK was aware of the high value that American culture places on competition as a means to bring out the best in people. I suspect that is why he told the following story.

TEACHING STORY: A TRUE VICTORY

Long ago there was an athletic competition in India similar to the Olympic games of today. Representatives were sent from all over the country to run a long distance. According to rules, everyone started at the same time. A throng of people surrounded the route and everyone debated who would prove the fastest.

Nearing the end of the race, there were only two contenders running neck in neck. Everyone wondered which one of these two, and therefore what region of the country, would be the winner. A short distance from the finish line, a heckler broke out of the crowd causing one of the two leading runners to fall down. After consulting the rules, the judges declared the runner who had crossed the finish line first to be the winner.

As the judges went to place a grand garland around his neck, the runner stepped back and would not accept the prize. "It is not right. My colleague fell down through no fault of his own, allowing me to win by chance. That is not a true victory." By this time, the runner who had fallen had gotten up and crossed the finish line second. Stepping forward, he replied, "I fell down through no fault of the victor. It was not his mistake. If anything, it is the result of my carelessness." The crowd gasped and grew silent as the judges consulted in a huddle. Raising his arms high, the head judge announced that the race would be run again in the morning with only these two participants.

The next day an even larger crowd gathered with everyone excited to watch the fastest runners in all of India. This time the runner who had fallen down the day before won by a step in a final dash to the finish line. Again, the judges lifted the grand garland and readied to place it upon the victor's neck, but he said, "I cannot accept the prize. My colleague beat me yesterday. Now we are only tied."

Again, the crowd gasped and the confused judges huddled. Then to the delight of everyone, a second garland was brought forth and both the runners were declared champions. While ancient, this story is still recounted because it reflects a competition that produced a true victory. Even if we don't want to do so, we all must compete in life. Yoga shows us how to bring forth our best and attain this kind of honest victory in which everyone wins.

AFTERWORD

Almost everyone spends the majority of their waking hours engaged in what we commonly call work. Life in the ashram was no different, except the communal context in which the work was performed encouraged residents to do it in the spirit of karma yoga. Its nomenclature reflected that intention. No one had a job in the ashram. Everyone had a seva, a position that enabled them to be of service.

In 1989, I was given a new seva in the resident business office. Personal computers were just coming into vogue, and one of my first assignments was to become proficient enough in word processing to create a template for a monthly resident newsletter. The design I came up with featured a short Swami Kripalu quote on the masthead. Below that was an attractively bordered open space for announcements, short articles, and information sharing. With the knowledge I'd gleaned from the software guide, that space could be formatted into a newspaper-like patchwork of text boxes and columns. Submitting a sample issue to my supervisor, I thought my task was done. A week later, I was called into the office of the department head to discuss it. Her name was Surabhi, someone I looked up to then, and still consider one of the best-ever ashram administrators.

Surabhi liked what I had done, but she had reservations about the SK quote. The sample I had come up with was fitting. A new one, however, would be needed every four weeks. She felt that it wasn't easy to distill a substantive spiritual teaching down to a soundbite. Including that as a design element might create a roadblock to getting the newsletter out on time. I acknowledged her concern, but it didn't occur to me as an obstacle. Opening my project file, I slid a page across the desk with six different quotes I had worked up as candidates for the mockup issue. "Here's a half years' worth," I said.

Surabhi put on a pair of reading glasses, and I sat quietly as she reviewed each one carefully. Having lived at the ashram when SK was in residence, Surabhi was steeped in his teachings. I got the feel that she was not about to allow anyone—especially a relatively new resident like me—to misconstrue them. As she put her glasses down, I didn't know what to expect until Surabhi's eyes brightened just a bit. She felt the topics I had chosen were pertinent to ashram life, and complimented my ability to get SK's points across so simply. I couldn't help but smile back when she ended her assessment by saying, "It seems you have a knack for this." Then came her decision. "If you are willing to do the quotes, along with everything else entailed in producing the newsletter, we can use this template." Only as I left her office did it dawn of me that getting permission to edit the ashram's namesake and founding yoga master was not a small thing.

You could draw a straight line from that meeting to the book you are holding in your hands. And that line extends to the concluding volume (forthcoming) in this trilogy: *Swami Kripalu's Ladder of Yoga*, which delves into my attempt to understand the significance of his teachings on postures, pranayama, and depth meditation and put them into practice. That book will begin with the following quote:

If humankind wants to rise above the darkness of ignorance to reach the light of knowledge, there is a need for a ladder. That ladder is yoga.

ACKNOWLEDGMENTS

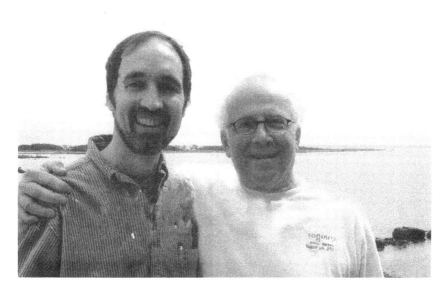

This book owes its existence to Justin Morreale, a dear friend and mentor who recognized the need to promote the teachings of Swami Kripalu during the decade he served as a leading member of Kripalu Center's board of trustees. While best known for his lengthy tenure as legal counsel to the Boston Red Sox, Justin is a devoted yogi. He started taking classes in 1970 and had twenty-five years of practice under his belt when he engineered a month away from his busy law firm in the summer of 1995 to become a Kripalu-certified teacher. Long before yoga was trendy, Justin pushed aside the tables of his conference room each week to guide an ever-changing cast of downtown Boston workers in postures, relaxation, and meditation. After seeing the need for this book,

Justin moved mountains to bring it into being by making a generous gift to Kripalu Center and galvanizing other donations to complete its funding. This charitable spirit has characterized his retirement years, during which he's played a leading role in a wealth of philanthropic endeavors doing incalculable good. Facing orthopedic health issues troublesome enough to sink anyone's spirits, he has remained active and cheerful by deepening his mantra and meditation practice. Justin embodies the ideal that SK held dear of being a socially-engaged yogi who energetically pursues his own work in the world while being a well-wisher of all. He has given me, and countless others, a shining example of a successful life rooted in-depth spirituality. This book is affectionately dedicated to Justin and his wife, Adele, with the prayer that any merit it generates comes back to them, their family, and their wide circle of friends as unsought grace. Additional acknowledgements will be included in the next and final installment of this grant-funded work.

APPENDIX 1

THE CHARACTER BUILDING PRINCIPLES OF YAMA AND NIYAMA

Although yama and niyama are only the first two stages of yoga, they contain the character building principles of every religion and approach to growth. Anyone who personifies an enormous power of purposeful determination is by necessity wedded to these principles. Master these virtues and you will not only excel in your chosen field of endeavor but become of benefit to the world.

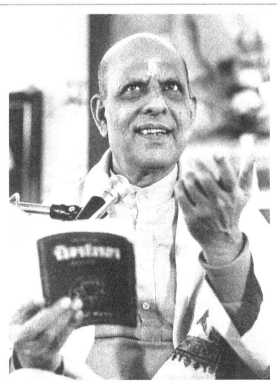

Swami Kripalu teaching from a yogic text.

It's impossible to say why Swami Kripalu left Bombay bound for America in the spring of 1977. Clearly, he was seeking a peaceful place entirely out of the public eye to complete his sadhana. But aiding the effort to transplant yoga in the West must also have factored into his thinking. When his plane touched down at JFK on May 20th, he was expected to resume the cloistered lifestyle he'd followed for over a quarter century. Yet he surprised everyone by setting aside his practice of mauna or silence for three months, delivering at least one and often two talks per day. The topic he returned to again and again in this series of informal discourses was the importance of yama and niyama.

Here is a distillation of how he defined and taught the twenty-three virtues he compiled from yoga's library of authoritative texts, drawn primarily from the content of those talks.

1. NON-VIOLENCE / AHIMSA

Nonviolence is always placed first among the spiritual disciplines. This foremost position signifies its primary importance. Indeed, a nonviolent disposition is the seed of genuine spirituality. When that seed sprouts, all the other disciplines come easily. This is why the practice of nonviolence is without equal; it is the superb religion for everyone.

In yoga, non-violence is called ahimsa which means non-harming. When one practices nonviolence, one refrains from causing distress in thought, word, or deed to any living creature.

Every person possesses the tendency toward violence to a greater or lesser extent. It's easy to think that nonviolence is not an issue for you. You never carry a knife in your pocket, or place a hatpin in your lapel. But it is a delusion to believe that violence is only committed by armed criminals and murderers.

A yogi knows that weapons come in two varieties, gross and subtle. Our thoughts can be like poison or nectar. The way in which we speak or write can bite another's heart. When angry, our temperament quickly turns cruel, and we assault even our loved ones with domineering actions and boisterous words. It is essential that we observe the discipline of nonviolence to purge ourselves of anger and hatred. Apathy in this discipline is the seat of violence. A yogi contemplates these matters deeply and adopts the ideal of nonviolence. Then by patiently and consistently allowing this ideal to guide and develop their life, he or she aspires to attain the most excellent expression of ahimsa, which is selfless love.

Stability of mind is essential in yoga sadhana. Ripples are produced when a stone, a pebble, or even sand grains fall into the still water of a lake surface. Similarly, all forms of violence generate mental disturbances, while true nonviolence is reflected in stillness and peace. Yet we are ordinary people and cannot practice true nonviolence right away. We must acknowledge that we lack this capacity, and remain vigilant in our efforts to refrain from violence and behave lovingly.

2. TRUTH / SATYA

The word satya or truth is ancient and has countless possible meanings. Today, I will discuss two aspects of satya vital to those practicing spiritual disciplines. The great masters of yoga realized the absolute truth. Nothing in the world perceived by our senses can match—in quality or quantity—the pure, unadulterated truth. This truth is the source of the entire universe; it is the ocean of existence itself. It is the divine truth that cannot be captured in language, and yet the beauty and profundity of it can be known. This requires us to close our ordinary eyes in meditation and break down the walls that block us from truth realization by opening the divine eye of samadhi.[1]

Intellectuals and spiritual teachers sometimes try to spread the truth by decorating it with various concepts. Everyone falls head over heels for this fancified truth, but still they remain stuck in their growth. A yogi who has gained the ability to be with the plain truth (the way things actually are) is more than courageous. Such a yogi is supremely valiant and assuredly moving from the darkness of ignorance to the light of truth.

Please remember that this stage of yoga can only be known by one willing to practice the ethical restraint of satya, which means truthfulness in speech. Here, satya is defined as speech that promotes the welfare of all living beings, and which is not mixed with untruth. Society is such that we have developed the habit from our earliest childhood of speaking untruth. Why do we find

---

[1] As this paragraph shows, SK used many different adjectives to point to the absolute truth at the causal core of reality, which the yoga tradition calls Brahman. Absolute truth is qualitatively different from the relative truth that we all recognize. When verbal statements match objective facts, they are said to be true. Similarly, when explanatory concepts and cognitive models of how things work display a close correspondence to reality, they are said to be true. These are examples of relative truth.

it so hard to speak truthfully? One important reason is that we have come to believe that truth is as worthless as a counterfeit coin and cannot help us get what we want in the world. Everyone accepts that we must speak untruth in order to get along in life and be happy. This firm belief that untruth is universally valuable leads us down the primrose path to falsehood.

Given this starting condition, we do not need at first to worry much about practicing truthfulness in speech. Instead, we should aim to merely delete a little from the mass of untruth we speak daily. Knowing how to speak means more than vocalizing vowels and consonants. It means more than being able to fill the air with eloquent but shallow talk. Unless we speak truthfully, speech is only noise.

Thought is the first stage of the speech process. What we call speech is correctly seen as verbalized thought. This is why a yogic aspirant who practices satya becomes more introspective, which leads them to naturally progress through the stages of self-observation, mental purification, character building, and meditation. Truthfulness in speech is like the fabled touchstone that turns everything it touches into gold. It can turn an ordinary seeker into an accomplished spiritual master. A yogi who has gained the ability to kindly speak truth and thereby transform enemies into loved ones has become fit to practice the meditations aimed at (absolute) truth realization.

3. NON-STEALING / ASTEYA

Non-stealing is a single discipline prescribed by the yogic scriptures, but it can be used to illustrate the relationship between yoga and morality. On close examination, it becomes obvious that all activities are performed through the medium of the mind. Tasks are easily grasped when the mind is clear, and the body works efficiently when the mind is peaceful. This explains why a degree of mental steadiness is essential to success in every field.

Yoga sadhana is also an activity, but one that requires special preparation because yoga cannot be effectively performed when the mind is agitated. This explains why anyone desiring to walk the path of yoga must practice morality. When we obtain what we need and want by honest means, our mind remains at peace. When we obtain what we desire by dishonest means, we invariably generate thoughts and feelings that disturb the mind and render progress in yoga impossible. Stealing is a form of violence, as it *always harms a victim. A thief must lie to conceal their theft. This shows how a single moral lapse can topple a whole fortress of spiritual disciplines.*

In yoga, non-stealing is defined as not desiring the wealth of another by thought, word or deed, and not taking anyone's possessions, no matter how small, without their permission. To put this definition into practice, a yogi must understand that material items are not the only things that can be stolen. For example, it is fine for a spiritual seeker to gather the good thoughts of inspiring orators and excellent authors. However, when speaking or writing those thoughts, they should acknowledge and express gratitude to the originator. Otherwise, they are stealing the work and fame of another. When a crow struts about wearing the feathers of a peacock, some form of theft has occurred.

Many people believe the world is a marketplace full of thieves. Master thieves are called aristocrats. Skilled thieves are called gentlemen. Only ordinary thieves are called criminals. In many ways, this commentary on society is correct. Despite the prevalence of poor conduct, a traveler on the path of yoga devotes themselves to virtuous conduct, and remains vigilant in the discipline of non-stealing.

4. MODERATION / BRAHMACHARYA

All my life, I have contemplated the subject of brahmacharya. Today I am only going to talk about its preliminary stage, which is a foundation of yogic practice.

Brahmacharya is a compound word in which "Brahma" is a reference to God and "charya" means "a vehicle in which to move." It can be literally defined as "the practice that carries you in the direction of the Lord." Many people think that brahmacharya is simply closing the sex door (celibacy), but its practice is broader than that.

Everyone today understands how a steam engine works. By bringing air, fire, and water together, steam energy is created. If that steam energy is properly contained in the boiler and mechanically channeled, it can accomplish tremendous things. Our body is not all that different. By bringing breath, food, and the digestive fire together, life energy is generated. Brahmacharya is the yogic practice of acting properly to create, contain, and channel that energy into good health and spiritual growth.

The best way to understand the basic practice of brahmacharya is to know the story of Lord Buddha. After long fasting, Buddha became weak and unable to stand. Seeing that he had gone too far, he discovered the path of moderation. Later Buddha taught this middle path by likening the body to a stringed instrument. If the strings are tightened too much, they break. If they are kept too loose, no sound comes forth. Only when the strings are moderately stretched do they sound the proper notes. Buddha knew that our body and mind are also an instrument. Anyone who wants to bring forth the music of happiness has to take the path of moderation.

Many people think that practicing brahmacharya is very difficult, but that is not true. All of us act in ways that protect our energy and health. This shows that everyone has a natural inclination toward brahmacharya. Yoga points out the need for right diet and regular exercise. It teaches us asanas to purify the body. It gives us virtues to contemplate to purify the mind. If you adopt these disciplines, and travel this path for a while, you will understand what brahmacharya is doing for you, and its practice will not seem overly difficult.

This much of a lesson on brahmacharya is enough for you today.

5. NON-ATTACHMENT / APARIGRAHA

To begin the practice of non-attachment, you must understand attachment and the teaching behind the word "parigraha," which means "to cling firmly to and accumulate." A baby recognizes his or her individual existence soon after birth. The moment the distinction of yours and mine arises in the mind, the seed of attachment takes root. By the time we are adults, several large cities could not contain everything we would like to have and hold onto if we had the power to do so.

Having accrued this mountain of attachments, non-attachment cannot be achieved in a single bound. Only a gradual, step-by-step approach is feasible. To take the first step, another Sanskrit term must be known. "Loka sangraham" means "to do things for the welfare of others." We all have experienced that there is a magic in mother's love. But what is it? Why does a school teacher solve a math problem on the blackboard? Does he solve it for himself? No, he solves it for the students. Acting to further our personal happiness is ordinary. Acting to benefit and give happiness to others is something beautiful, and a step in the direction of non-attachment. This is why yoga considers any actions not motivated by selfish ends and done to promote the public welfare, express a genuine love of humanity, or serve the Lord, to be a form of non-attachment. Such actions are true social work, which can only be performed by one intentionally or unconsciously embarked on the path of non-attachment.

The next step is to cultivate a voluntary simplicity in living. One discharges his or her duties, while remaining self-aware and free of obsessive desires. Living this way, we gradually see that happiness does not come from the material objects we've collected, all our memories of past enjoyments that we would like to repeat, or fulfilling our dreams for the future. Realizing this, our behavior changes gradually, and we are able to drop our desires one by one.

The non-attachment of an advanced yogi is qualitatively different from the non-attachment of a developing yogi. This is reflected in the word "aparigraha," which is the antonym of "parigraha." It means to "firmly let go" and "be unattached from everything." This condition can only be achieved by learning how to detach your attention from the activity of the mind and senses through the process of yoga. For this to happen, you must enjoy and attach yourself to the practice of introspective meditation with the same strength as you were formerly attached to the sensuous things of the world.

This higher form of non-attachment is born when a yogi observes their thoughts and feelings as a witness and refrains from being moved by them. It attains maturity only when the yogi gains the ability to fixate attention on their object of meditation in dharana. Until then, a person should remain content practicing aparigraha in whatever form is possible for them in their current life circumstances, allowing their character to gradually develop until the penance of yogic non-attachment grows appealing.

6. PURIFICATION / SAUCHA

The Sanskrit word saucha means "purity" or "purification." In yoga, there are two types of saucha: physical and mental, with each one having an internal and external aspect.

Everyone should bathe daily to keep the pores open and help the skin do its work as an organ of perspiration and elimination. Knowing this, the ancient rishis cleansed the exterior of their bodies by rubbing the skin with dirt to remove excess oils, and afterward bathing in water. While I was growing up, most Indians bathed three times a day in a sincere attempt to continue this practice. But the baths they took were only rituals in which they poured a bowl or two of water over their head and trunk. In terms of yoga, they were not practicing saucha of the body. Anyone rubbing the skin of such a person would probably remove layers and layers of dirt.

Today we have many conveniences in our homes and cleanse ourselves with luxurious toiletries. Yet the most useful substances for cleaning the body remains water and soap. While important, bathing only cleanses the exterior of the body. A truly pure body is only obtained by one who eats moderately, exercises regularly to efficiently digest their food, and evacuates their bowels properly to keep the intestines free of accumulated fecal matter. All these internal things are necessary to inhabit a pure physical body that radiates health and the absence of disease.

Saucha also includes cultivating a wholesome and pure mind. Our mind is an ocean of thoughts. We have a greater chance to evolve if it contains more positive than negative thoughts, and suffer a greater risk of deteriorating if it contains more negative than positive thoughts. We are all highly influenced by our environment and the countless people surrounding us, from which both positive and negative thoughts are generated. Positive thinking is nourished by inspirational reading, prayer, and meditation. This explains why the yogic texts advise one to frequent good company, avoid bad company, and study the scriptures to purify the mind. Mental purity is reflected externally in loving speech and virtuous conduct. Internally, it is the pure intention that underlies and motivates such actions.

Our mind is always in motion and radiates thoughts like the rays of the sun. Most people are not aware that they are continually transmitting their thoughts and also receiving the thoughts of others. But an advanced yogi can see this exchange in minute detail. We all know that different electrical frequencies can be transmitted and received via signals from a radio station. When the mental instrument is highly purified by yoga sadhana, the transmitting and receiving centers of the mind work readily together to facilitate non-verbal communication by the conscious exchange of thoughts.

7. CONTENTMENT / SANTOSH

Today I will talk about the niyama of contentment, which in Sanskrit is called santosh. Santosh is noteworthy among the niyamas because contentment and its opposite—discontent—are both useful to the yogi. If we understand the appropriate role of each, we become able to digest and progress from all of our life experiences.

A content individual has the capacity to bear the difficulties and problems of life while remaining optimistic and happy. Most of us are discontent. We are always unhappy with our present state and live with a dream of future fulfillment. This manner of thinking keeps us eager to escape our current circumstances. We neglect to gratefully acknowledge all that we have in hopes of getting more. Even when good fortune comes our way, we do not pause to experience contentment, but choose instead to strive for more gain. People with this mindset possess a little bit of contentment and a boatload of discontentment.

The needs of a person who values contentment are relatively few because contentment renders the mind steady and is its own source of happiness. Joyfully accepting whatever life provides, they do not hanker after more than is at hand. After making efforts that bring genuine material or spiritual progress, a person with this mindset enjoys the fulfillment that naturally follows. It is in this sense that contentment is a true virtue. Yet the niyama of santosh does not mean that its opposite is of no value.

A yogi inclined toward santosh should pay attention to any discontent felt within. A yogi intends to grow. Spiritually and also materially, they want to make real progress. Some dissatisfaction is necessary to do this; it gives us the inspiration to make an effort to go further. It is through this form of discontent that a wise person awakens, becomes devoted to their work, and grows increasingly enthusiastic, skillful, faithful, courageous, patient, and self-controlled. This form of discontentment is indeed an auspicious sign of future victory. Conversely, if your practice of contentment is producing a diminished effort, unskilled work, apathy, laziness, faithlessness, impatience, and intolerance, it is not santosh but a sign that your journey of growth has ended. When the niyama of santosh is understood properly, a yogi sees that contentment is a fulfilled state of mind, and discontent is one of the aids to attaining it.

I will conclude this lecture by telling you an important truth. In order to know true contentment, you must be making an effort to progress toward what you most want in life. Otherwise, all your efforts to alleviate discontent will come from a state of helplessness. My experience is that yoga is like a store that doesn't deliver. If you call the store, you get the warehouse and will be told that there's a big stock of contentment with your name on it, but you have to come and get it yourself. It is my prayer and blessing that you seek out and receive this true contentment.

8. AUSTERITY / TAPAS

The term tapas is profound. It has an ordinary meaning that can be understood by everyone. It also has an extraordinary meaning that can only be understood by a practicing yogi.

The ordinary meaning of tapas is "discipline," and in particular "the self-discipline required to be consistent in a practice." Don't believe that only great yogis can do tapas. Research scientists are also tapasvins (practitioners of tapas). First, they must dedicate themselves to learning everything there is to know about one field of study. Only then can they employ the disciplines of science to answer a question that adds to our collective knowledge. Without this ordinary kind of tapas, making the journey of either science or yoga is impossible. Every yogic aspirant needs the self-discipline required to regularly do techniques to uplift their health and gain spiritual knowledge.

Tapas also means "to generate light or heat." This is a reference to the psychic energy generated by the practice of yogic disciplines. Just as a hot fire smelts impure ore into gold, the energy of tapas purifies the seeker. In practice, the word "tapas" is best defined as "austerity" because it describes the extraordinary mindset of a yogi who is willing to undergo this smelting process to purify their body, mind, and speech.

There are many forms of tapas, each of which requires the yogi to practice self-restraint. Fasting or eating only what is necessary to sustain health is a powerful bodily tapas. So is the practice of celibacy. Observing a vow of silence is a tapas that quickly straightens out our crooked speech. Reciting mantra or curbing the flow of thought in meditation is a tapas that purifies the mind. Any specific form of tapas will also have a general effect of increasing a yogi's spiritual radiance.

Without a willingness to pass through the fire of tapas, the character cannot be remolded. But observing a yogic tapas is not the same as engaging in some unthinking austerity such as whipping yourself or lying on a bed of nails. A spiritual discipline should not harm the body or mind. Tapas is not self-mortification, which only insults the body and makes the mind dull. Tapas is self-purification, which always leads to the sweetening of speech and the brightening of body, mind, and heart. A true yogi yearns to become the light, and is willing to burn until their soul remains perpetually lit. It is this state of voluntary burning that is tapas. Its purest form is an abiding love for God or Truth and unyielding desire to know the highest through yoga sadhana.

9. SELF-STUDY / SVADHYAYA

"Svadhyaya" is a compound word. Sva means "self" or atman. Adhyaya means "to study." A yogic aspirant practices svadhyaya to get to know their true self.

The great acharyas of the past were masterful teachers. Knowing that it was not possible for an aspirant to practice the advanced form of svadhyaya right away, they developed beginning and intermediate steps. A beginning aspirant practiced mantra japa, meditatively reciting a word, meaningful phrase, or name of the Lord in which they had faith. We all understand how laundry detergent can be used to clean clothes. Japa is much like a washing machine in which the detergent of a mantra is used to cleanse the mind of impure and distracting thoughts.

Mantra japa renders the mind fit for the intermediate step of scripture study. Humankind is very old. During its time on earth, our forebears faced countless problems. Whenever solutions were found, they were written into texts considered sacred to pass down those solutions to future generations. This treasury of knowledge collected by our ancestors is available to any person who can read these texts with that understanding. But today our definition of scripture can be broadened to include any text of true spiritual wisdom, whether ancient or not. An intermediate aspirant reads and reflects upon one or more of these texts to inform their view of life and the path ahead.

While the knowledge gained from scripture study is only inferential, it prepares an aspirant to practice true svadhyaya. This means to search for an experiential answer to an essential philosophical question. Who am I? What am I? What is the nature of this Self? How did this whole universe come to be and what is my place in it? Is there a Supreme Being or Ultimate Reality and, if so, how can it be known? Answers to questions like these cannot be realized by thinking. We must study the self directly. This requires us to introvert the attention through contemplation, and descend into the depths of the mind through meditation, in search of a real resolution.

Lord Buddha is famous for asserting, "Yes, there is a solution to suffering, and I have realized it." Like Buddha and all the yogis of old, we must remain steadfast in our journey of svadhyaya. Now, I am not advising you to become a seeker of liberation like me. I am only telling you to pursue svadhyaya until you can say, "Yes, I have found a way to live as myself that brings me security, enjoyment, and genuine contentment." Yet this trio of mantra japa, scripture study, and meditative svadhyaya can be continued. It can carry a dedicated practitioner all the way to a realization that dissolves away their deepest human dilemmas. But completing this journey inevitably requires spiritual passion, persistence, and courage. It would not be right for me to give you false inspiration. Take refuge in the foundational practices and find out if you truly desire to travel further. If so, seek to hear the deeper teachings straight from the mouth of an experienced acharya. That is the proven pathway to becoming a high caliber practitioner of svadhyaya.

10. SURRENDER TO THE LORD / ISHVARA PRANIDHANA

It is not right to look at Ishvara Pranidhana as merely one of the niyamas. It is a core component of any form of yoga and must be understood in that context. Let's begin by examining the word surrender, which in yoga can be defined as "voluntarily taking refuge in something more powerful than yourself."

In the stories of ancient India, a king whose army had been defeated in battle would often have to surrender to another king whose army proved victorious. But this type of surrender was neither attractive nor accepted by the yogis. A helpless king surrendering by necessity to a vanquishing enemy would likely have hatred in his heart. A yogic aspirant who takes refuge in a universal force does so willingly with a heart full of love. Such an aspirant has not been defeated; they are aligning with an all-powerful force.

Various schools of yoga envision what this niyama calls "the Lord" differently. It might be seen as the essential Self (atman), or the macrocosmic Brahman. It might be seen as the Truth or the divine intelligence informing nature. It might be seen as the Supreme Being or a particular form of God. All these are equal terms to be applied in one and the same practice of surrender.

Before we can surrender to any of these, we have to make contact with whatever it is that we take as the highest. It is a psychological principle that we can trust completely only when we are convinced that what we are surrendering to holds the place of the supreme. This requires more than belief, faith, or deep thinking. It is a matter of direct experience. In order to establish this contact, we have to practice the limbs of yoga. We have to use the yogic techniques to disconnect from the senses, cutting off all the other contacts and attachments that keep the mind disturbed. When this contact is made, the practice of Ishvara Pranidhana becomes possible and starts to occur naturally.

Hearing this you might ask, "Please tell us what surrender to the Lord means for a novice spiritual aspirant?" Ishvara Pranidhana is ordinarily defined in religious terms as "dedicating your actions and all their consequences to the Lord." At first, only those actions performed to purify the body and mind, worship one's chosen deity, or serve humanity are considered Ishvara Pranidhana. For example, actions performed simply to obtain money or gain recognition are not included. Similarly, just eating is not considered Ishvara Pranidhana. But eating after praying, "Oh Lord, I'm taking this food with gratitude and faith that it will sustain my body and purify my mind so I can progress upon the pilgrimage of my life" can rightly be considered an act dedicated to the Lord.

As novices, we have limited capacity and must be content to take small steps. We should avoid harmful actions and do all the good things that enable us to grow beyond a narrow selfishness. By surrendering even a little to ideals like these, we will receive inspiration and make steady progress until we begin to see that all our actions spring from the same spiritual source. It is at this stage of practice that Ishvara Pranidhana becomes essential to yoga. Afterward, unless one is growing in a chosen form of surrender, their yoga sadhana comes to a halt.

The Almighty is the true friend of all. Can friendship be possible between a human being and the infinite and omnipotent? Although friends need not be equal, they must have love for each other. Love is the very root of friendship. If this type of love for God or Truth arises in the heart of a yogic aspirant, it will generate a force that will continually lead in the direction of Ishvara Pranidhana. Everything needed will happen naturally, and the aspirant will feel that nothing need be done willfully, or even thought about.

11. FORBEARANCE / KSHAMA

Each day we cross paths with countless people whose behavior affects us. It is natural to feel aggravated by those who knowingly or unknowingly do unpleasant things. Many of us can simply ignore the slight of a first-degree offense. Some of us can tolerate the pain of a second-degree violation by suppressing our anger and restraining the desire to punish the offender. Few if any of us can tolerate a high crime of the third-degree without giving vent to our animosity. We unconsciously strike back because our intellect ceases to function and defensive instincts take over whenever we are sufficiently provoked.

The great yogis of the past were aware of these natural responses. Yet they still included forbearance in their list of niyamas and defined it as "refraining from the projection of aversion to any living beings regardless of how they behave." That's because they saw that aversion, animosity, and hatred are thought forms that violently agitate the mind and steal away our peace and happiness. With aggravations bound to occur, the only way to prevent these disturbances is to cultivate an attitude of forbearance. Aggressive actions are like a sword. Where responding to anger with anger almost always causes a war to break out, raising the shield of forbearance can foil the blow without generating a swordfight.

The ability to restrain and not feed the fire of immediate anger against the offender is the first step in forbearance. Consistency in yoga practice is an unfailing way to gain this ability to objectively witness such powerful thoughts and feelings. After that, do not allow disrespect, hatred, or other forms of ill will toward the offender to lodge and multiply in the mind. Entertain only those thoughts, words, and deeds that lessen mental disturbance. If necessary, the attention can be deliberately turned away from the immediate situation and placed upon some interesting and pacifying subject.

Only those aspirants who genuinely understand the importance of maintaining mental steadiness and overcoming our violent nature can implement these steps in formidable circumstances. The average person succumbs to the situation, in part because they do not fully understand the harm caused by roiling the mind with anger. Sometimes it is said, "The mind is not a goat that can be tamed by anyone. It is a lion that can be tamed only by a truly courageous person." This is why forbearance is considered a niyama; it is an austerity without which the lasting happiness born of a peaceful mind cannot be attained.

You may think this analysis of forbearance is useful only for householders practicing yoga in society. Renunciates live in seclusion aloof from these kinds of difficulties. But this is not the case. To illustrate my point, picture me on an airplane flying from India to America. The gentleman sitting next to me starts smoking a cigar. Since I do not smoke, I cannot tolerate the smoke. And yet, I must tolerate it. In addition, the brother sitting across the aisle is eating meat and drinking liquor, which he thoroughly enjoys because of the odors. Not liking the sight or smells, I must bear my feelings of disgust.[2]

The brother eating is sensitive enough to say, "Swamiji, please excuse me for consuming liquor and meat." Through this simple apology, an intolerable situation becomes somewhat tolerable. Thus, I am able to reply, "Please do not hesitate on my part, sir. One must accept such things while traveling."

But not everyone takes the emotional reactions of others into consideration. The smoker's habit generates overpowering desires in him, and he says nothing. Perhaps he thinks, "Smoking is allowed on this airplane. Why should I stop, just because some swami is sitting near me? What's wrong with smoking anyhow?" Abandoning the question of whether his actions are proper or improper, it is best for me to divert my attention elsewhere.

Forbearance should not be thought of as merely a tool to cope with social injustices. The person behaving unkindly is often a relative or loved one. Moreover, we ourselves will commit wrongs that require the forbearance of others. Nor should we feel smug if by chance we have forgiven someone once, twice, or three times. Nor should we practice forbearance within a select group. Everyone must be forgiven. The one and only way to fill our lives with happiness is to empty them of anger and judgment by generously distributing forbearance to everyone. Practiced in this manner, forbearance is an affectionate mother destined to give birth to genuine compassion (daya).

12. STEADFASTNESS / DHRITI

Dhriti means to be steadfast and is defined as holding firmly to a chosen course of action all the way to completion. Regardless of whether seeking to advance outwardly or inwardly, a yogic aspirant must gain this ability to make a clear commitment and carry it out with firm determination. Steady, stable, decisive, resolute, self-composed, these are all qualities associated with dhriti.

It is mistaken to imagine yogic dhriti as strength of willpower alone, which often by itself proves weak. Dhriti is an application of all our faculties. A clear and resolute choice to undertake a defined task brings mental steadiness. Steadiness reins in the senses and gives birth to a calm patience.

---

[2] The record reflects that SK refrained from eating for the duration of this trip. Fasting is known to heighten the sense of smell and increase emotional lability, which adds context to this story

Patiently practicing yoga techniques awakens sleeping energies. Energy brings forth courage and the fortitude to persevere through difficulties. Dhriti is all of these working powerfully together to generate skillful action and arrive at the desired result.

A novice yogi learns the principles of dhriti and applies them to advance outwardly in life. An intermediate yogi uses dhriti to perform the highly desirable actions of yama and niyama. In yama, it means firmly letting go of harmful actions. In niyama, this means holding firmly onto beneficial actions. Both are required to develop the character. An advanced yogi has attained the degree of dhriti (the yogic stage of dharana) required to enter the mysteries of yoga sadhana. At all these stages, aspirants practice the same dhriti but to different degrees. Yet the dhriti of all these aspirants is not the same as the dhriti of one who has reached the far shore of yoga. The indomitable conviction of such a soul is extraordinary in every respect.

The Bhagavad Gita tells us the intellect of most people is fickle. As a result, a resolute decision cannot be reached and dhriti remains impossible. In order to escape this limbo of indecisiveness, the niyama of mati must be adopted. These two—dhriti and mati—walk hand in hand and must be learned and practiced together.

13. DECISIVENESS / MATI

The primary function of the intellect is to make decisions. Mati is the discipline of steadying the mind so the intellect can generate firm decisions made with potent conviction. This type of decisive intellect is needed to walk the path of yoga.

We must understand that there are good reasons why some of our resolutions get followed up by action and some fall by the wayside. There is a logic to this that can be followed to produce firm decisions. This is one of the light-giving secrets of yoga, and an aspirant aided by the logic of mati no longer wanders in the dark.

We are all familiar with the opposite of mati, which is a wavering and fickle mind. Some commentators say all our wavering is caused by doubt and fear. We doubt that we have made the right decision, and we fear that it will not bring the desired results. For example, imagine that you do not know if an expensive piece of jewelry is brass or gold. If it is only brass, you will pay too much. If it is gold, you will miss an opportunity for profit. Until this doubt is resolved, you cannot make the purchase or walk away. Your fearful mind wavers, and on the level of action you remain in limbo.

Yoga accepts that fear and doubt play a role in the mind's wavering, but it considers the matter with greater subtlety. Our minds have grown accustomed to being restless. As a result, the intellect makes decisions too quickly. To make matters worse, decisions are repeatedly made and unmade. We are unable to rely on a decision, because it is apt to be revisited and replaced by another and different decision. Consequently, the restless mind oscillates back and forth, we make many mistakes, and tend to leave challenging tasks incomplete. The Bhagavad Gita tells us that victory in life and yoga sadhana are only gained by a yogi firm in their decisions and determined to act skillfully. If this is correct, what can be done?

First, we must realize that if our decisions are hastily made they will not last long. Our minds are well-aware of all our past experiences. To make a firm decision, the problem at hand must be studied carefully. As long as the situation is not pondered deeply, the mind's doubts will remain and arriving at a thoughtful decision is impossible. We must grow used to contemplating our decisions carefully. This can only be done when the mind is calm. We should not be swayed by superficial inspiration, regardless of how impressed we are by alluring ideas and promises of easy success. Impulsive choices born from excited mind states prove weak and do not lead to accomplishment, so decision-making should be postponed until favorable conditions exist.

While contemplating a decision, we must take into consideration the necessity of following through on it and cultivate a strong desire to see it to completion. Challenges and obstacles must be foreseen. A decision should not be made until we have complete faith in our ability to carry it out despite any difficulties we may face.

After a decision is made, we should expect fears and doubts to arise. When trying to accomplish something truly difficult that we earnestly desire, this may produce painful and hard-to-ignore projections. Yet this should not lead us to change a correct decision. If, after calm contemplation, a course of action needs to be reconsidered, that should be consciously decided. Otherwise, we should proceed using the situation as an opportunity to strengthen our faith.

Yoga teaches that the soul lies deep in the center of the mental mechanism. It is said that anyone able to touch into the soul can have all their wishes fulfilled. This is because the soul's wishes are unfailingly proper, and always accompanied by a firm determination to realize them. Until we reach this *level, we should cultivate dhriti and mati to obtain the complete form of yogic willpower. That willpower should only be used to pursue our rightful desires, especially the desire to undertake the disciplines prescribed to realize the soul and achieve the lasting peace unrelated to the fulfillment of any desire. A yogi illumines the mind to discover the brilliant beam of Truth itself.*

14. PATIENCE / DHAIRYA

Recently we've discussed the mental disciplines of forbearance, steadfastness, and decisiveness in promoting steadiness and preserving peace of mind. Intrinsic to the practice of all such disciplines is another niyama that yoga calls dhairya or patience, which I will talk about today.

We all have patience—to a greater or lesser degree. Examining the degree to which we have patience can teach us an important lesson. Patience can be defined as the capacity to remain mentally steady and productively focused on a task despite the arising of distractions and difficulties. When the mind reaches its limit and abandons patience, it becomes completely restless. This results in a cascade of emotions on a spectrum from anger to depression. Harmful or unproductive actions may be taken in anger. Depression may cause a person to become apathetic and inactive. All of this is known to the science of psychology.

When patience is lost, happiness itself is lost, because happiness cannot be separated from its constituents of mental peace and steadiness. Along with present happiness, an opportunity for accomplishment has also been lost, as setbacks have not strengthened but toppled one's steadiness of mind, requiring it to be rebuilt. Worse yet, a person unable to accomplish an important task may consider themselves a failure, creating a dark impression in the mind likely to impede future happiness. This clearly demonstrates how impatience brings defeat. This explains the Indian adage, "Those who wish to be successful must take refuge in patience." When the mind wavers and gives in to impatience in the very moments that could precede success, it is like a ship sinking within eyesight of the shore.

All of us begin life impulsive and impatient. But these are qualities we give up as we mature. Many of us grow to an average level of patience, but we do not have to stop there. Walking the path of yoga, one's capacity for forbearance, steadfastness, decisiveness, and patience can continually develop. Enthusiasm increases as these virtues are understood and practiced.

Impulsivity is gradually replaced by stability. Persistence and purposefulness gain sway as mental steadiness is established.

But cultivating patience itself requires patience. In India, many mango trees require twelve years to mature, after which they produce abundantly. Be aware of this fact, and don't allow impatience to cut down your mango tree of patience after one, two, or even eleven years of practice. Exercise patience by allowing whatever time is needed for your practice of these niyamas to bear fruit.

15. COMPASSION / DAYA

A person flourishes when they are continually using their life circumstances to develop good character. In yoga, character is built brick-by-brick through the disciplines of yama and niyama. But to use the word "discipline" shows that we've been using the perspective of jnana and karma yoga in which character is built through understanding and right action. But the bhakti yoga path of love and devotion can yield the same results. How can this be so?

Forbearance and the ability to forgive come naturally to a loving person, as does a special type of steadfastness that expresses as a dedication to the well-being of their loved ones. A loving person is patient, and a patient mind is able to contemplate and draw subtle distinctions, which imbues their decisions with wisdom. The heart of a loving person is full of pure intentions, which makes them straightforward, free of deviousness, and charitably disposed. There is only one yoga, but it is important to understand how the pure character sought through study (jnana yoga) and right action (karma yoga) can also be gained by love and devotion (bhakti yoga). In truth, elements from all these paths (knowledge, discipline, love) must come together to sculpt the character of a great spiritual master.

Today I will expound upon one of the bhakti niyamas called "daya" or "compassion." Daya can also be defined as kindness, empathy, being merciful, or well-wishing. In all this world, there is not a single human being who does not have pain. From this perspective, we live in an ocean of suffering. This is why some yogic texts declare the true name of this world is "the abode of pain."

Yet even in this weakness, where we ourselves are in misery and deserving of compassion, we can choose to show compassion to others. This is a unique response to human life, and one that provides us a special strength. A person who develops this strength fully, and gives mercy freely without any desire for their own gain or aggrandizement, ceases to be an average person eligible for compassion and is transformed into an ocean of compassion itself.

The pain of others does not touch everyone. Daya begins simply as an outgrowth of caring and must spring from a genuine desire to eradicate or mitigate the misery of others. Upon seeing a suffering person, the onlooker's heart melts. Empathy arises in their mind, accompanied by the motivation to extend help. At this stage, the pain of another has become one's own. Through this, the flame of compassion has been kindled.

The realm for extending love is great. Not only the impoverished and disadvantaged need compassion. The wealthy and privileged are beset by suffering too. Indeed, all living beings are worthy of compassion. Those who are sightless, immobile, deaf, and infirm can extend especially tender feelings of empathy and mercy. The pilgrimage into this realm of love is an auspicious one, as extending compassion only begins as a sympathetic act. By removing all the blocks to our growth, this single quality of daya becomes the cause of many virtues and divine qualities in us.

Sometimes this progression is expressed poetically. It's said that Ahimsa gives birth to a lovely daughter named Compassion, whose nature is to extend mercy. By following her nature, Ahimsa's daughter grows into the radiant Goddess of Compassion, who showers her grace upon everyone unconditionally and engenders the happiness of all.

16. STRAIGHTFORWARDNESS / ARJAVA

Among the lesser known niyamas is one called arjava, which can be translated as straightforwardness. While different definitions of the term may be offered, the guiding idea is to conduct yourself in a way that is simple, natural, upright, and truthful. To do what is simple and natural sounds easy, but one practicing arjava quickly sees how this is not the case.

The family is the cradle for human development, and children are often raised in environments that do not invite straightforwardness. A parent may frequently say things that deceive their innocent son or daughter in minor ways, not out of selfishness, but with good intentions and a desire to protect them. The child soon recognizes that mother and father also relate to one another in this way. At first, a child mirrors back these deceptions in small acts, telling what are called "white lies" that sugar coat the truth.

Engaging in this game, they cease being simple and straightforward, projecting an image to court approval.

This is understandable, as a child born into such an environment would not thrive in any other way. As this tendency grows, the maturing child may never consider that anything wrong is being done. Yet a pattern of artifice has spread throughout their character, which is reinforced when even friends and well-wishers deceive them with the flower petals of flattery. This picture that I am painting is so prevalent that it is rare to find anyone nowadays who is simple, real, and truthful.

Understanding the origin of our crookedness, a special effort is required to remove it and regain our innocence. This is best done in proper sequence. First, the deviousness and cunning of our thinking must be acknowledged and renounced. Next, the distortions of our speech must be recognized and removed with the practice of satya (truth). As these steps are taken, our actions will become increasingly free of artifice. This practice must be carried out until arjava becomes an attitude that pervades the mind and ego.

The scriptures say that realization comes naturally to the straightforward aspirant. At this time, when society as a whole has lost sight of the importance of ethical principles, it is enough for us as individuals to accept the need for simplicity, naturalness, and truthfulness. Renouncing cunning and artifice, our relations with others will grow harmonious and our progress on the spiritual path quicken.

17. MODERATION IN DIET / MITAHAR

The term mitahar is composed of two words. Mit means moderate and ahar means food. Many people believe that eating moderately means taking a fixed, small quantity of food per day, but this is mistaken. The appetite of young children impels continual nibbling since their bodies are growing. Adolescents require even more food to fuel growth spurts. Similarly, pregnant and nursing women have special needs. On days adults exercise little, their appetite is naturally reduced. On days they exercise a lot, more food is needed. Elderly people tend to be less active and thus eat less. In much the same way that the diet of an ant and an elephant are altogether different, what is normal for one person is not normal for another.

Mitahar can be defined as "eating the precise amount of food required to keep the body alert and operating efficiently." What this means in practice can be stated simply—not too much, and not too little—but moderation is easier said than done. If a delicious dish is placed in front of an orator while they are preaching about the virtue of mitahar, they will want to stop their sermon until the food has been eaten. Wise men and women are similarly hampered because the lust for food is controlled by the tongue as much as the mind. This path of mitahar is so slippery that even advanced yogis routinely slide off it. This difficulty is a secret we keep to ourselves. Who would want to admit our gluttonous lower natures publicly?

In India, the topic of moderation in diet has been given deep consideration. Countless experiments have been conducted by its inquisitive sages. Indian religion as a whole accepts that mitahar plays a vital role in spiritual life because a person's energy is generated and maintained by right diet. Among the three principal religions, Jainism emphasizes the practice of fasting, which purifies the body quickly but requires suppression. And after fasting, one's old patterns of eating often resume. Buddhism and Sanatana Dharma (yoga) emphasize moderation in diet, which maintains the health of the body through the exercise of discrimination and restraint. Through mitahar, we can gradually achieve a level of physical purity that can be sustained.

Life eventually teaches us that when we eat too much, too often, with too little discrimination, we overburden the digestive system. Not only does our stomach hurt, but we open the door to disease. In times of illness, mother nature may intervene. She takes away our appetite to give our digestive system a rest. Periodic fasting cleanses the system and is a good way to reset our taste buds and regain self-control. But fasting alone is not an effective strategy. Eventually, the wisdom of learning to limit the amount we eat to remain healthy, rather than overeating and becoming a victim of disease, becomes obvious. The time is now ripe to take up the niyama of mitahar.

I am speaking to you as an old sanyasi (renunciate yogi). For many years, I've taken only one meal a day, but that does not mean it has been easy for me to practice mitahar. In India, my devotees were always bringing me a variety of foods including all of my favorite dishes. Even if I ate a little bit of everything, it still got to be too much. Periodically, I would have to fast. At 65 years, God has given me some wisdom, and my mind is not as mischievous as earlier in my life. In America, I've made arrangements that no spare food is kept in my residence. One meal of simple foods is brought to me each day. I've accepted the fact that a yogi has to practice moderation in diet in order to have the energy to keep growing toward liberation. I am saying this so you can learn from my experience, even at this late stage of my practice, and understand the discipline of mitahar further.

For a practitioner of yoga, food should be taken with humility, reverence, and gratitude. Eating a digestible and tasty meal that fills the stomach one half with food, one quarter with water, and leaves one quarter empty for the circulation of the vital air—this is the scriptural definition of mitahar. For the yogi, regulating food in this way is observed as a great vow. If a yogi eats moderately, it is not necessary to fast. Truly, one who can practice restraint while eating without suppression can rightly be considered a great yogi.

It's easy for a wise person to sit down for a meal and lose all discrimination or even turn into a ravenous animal. While trying to retain my discrimination, I often call to mind a scriptural verse, "One practicing mitahar in the end proves victorious."

18. FAITH / ASTIKYA

Today I will talk to you about the niyama of astikya. The English word faith has many meanings. It can refer to the religion to which a person subscribes, or their firm belief in its tenets based on the authority of its founders. This is different from the niyama of astikya as taught by the science of yoga.

Astikya begins at the level of psychology. Psychologists know that every action we take is motivated by a type of faith based on our past experiences. When an action produces a successful result, it strengthens the faith that motivated it. When an action fails, it weakens the faith that motivated it. Seen in this way, the faith motivating our actions is continually developing as it is either reinforced or destroyed in the learning process of life.

We are constantly taking action, and it might seem that everyone should quickly gain the experience and faith required to accomplish their aims and desires. However, our minds are filled with past impressions. Some of these are positive impressions that reinforce useful behaviors. But others are negative impressions at the root of our destructive traits and self-sabotaging habits. Unless we have the steadfastness to carry out positive actions until they yield success, we are subject to lassitude, doubt, and discouragement. When such thoughts and patterns arise, we are likely to abandon our right actions through faithlessness. This is why the first task of a spiritual aspirant is to examine both the positive and negative impressions that influence their mental state and cultivate the strong faith that is the foundation of accomplishment.

To not just develop psychologically but also evolve spiritually, a person has to perform many actions that are totally new. Where do we get the motivation to do something completely new and novel? In yoga, it is said that there are two sources. The first is to have faith in your guru (teacher) and the disciplines prescribed by the scriptures to advance you on the spiritual path. The second is to trust the stream of ideas and knowings coming from the intuitive mind, where the seeds of many subtle actions are waiting to sprout at the first opportunity. These new actions are like a fire that burns away old conceptions so fresh experience, knowledge, and motivation can come forth.

The disciplines of yama and niyama are scientifically designed to bring health, happiness, and accomplishment. Only by conducting the experiment of yoga can you gain the level of astikya (verified faith) required to persevere in their practice. This kind of faith is self-nourishing and never defeated. Facing failure, it becomes increasingly aware, enthusiastic, and aligned with dharma. If one action does not succeed, it tries another. And if that action fails, it tries a third. In the same way that butter is obtained from the process of churning, all these determined actions purify the body and mind. This process brings more than success. For one remaining faithful, the knowledge of yoga (direct experience of unity consciousness) is gained solely by intuition. Spontaneously and automatically, it just comes out from within.

19. CHARITY / DANA

Human life is fraught with problems. As soon as an old problem dissolves, a new one arises to take its place. Given this state of affairs, it is wise to focus on resolving the root problems from which countless difficulties and dilemmas sprout. For example, a wife might tell her husband, "We have to pay the rent. How are we going to also buy the clothes, food, and schooling needed by our children?" While each of these matters is different, the root problem is singular. All these questions will evaporate the moment enough money is obtained.

Indeed, the question of material abundance is a root problem of life. In India, many wrongfully take sanyas (renounce the world) in order to secure a supply of free food from equally poor householders. One primary definition of yoga is "skillfulness in action." It is through the correct practice of yoga (skillful action) and dharma (right way of living) that individuals can prosper.

Yet the sages have also taught that one facet of this dharma is the niyama called "dana" or charity. Dana is setting aside a bit of whatever you receive and giving it away with compassionate feelings to benefit others who are also deserving but in circumstances that leave them in need of assistance.

In ancient India, every element of dharma was believed to possess scientific validity. The yogic sages observed that the universe is exceedingly generous. When a farmer sows one seed, a plant comes forth that produces thousands of seeds. To enjoy abundance, the instruction of these sages was to put this universal principle into practice. Whatever you receive, share a portion with others. By establishing yourself in the flow of generosity, whatever you give will come back many-fold.

In modern times, we can see that it is irrational to conflate wealth and prosperity. A rich person who is not generous is not really wealthy, because they feel and behave like a pauper. Conversely, those who are poor but generous are actually wealthy, because they feel and behave like a rich person. Even today, cultured people follow the advice of the sages by first dedicating their earnings to meet the needs of their family, then donating a portion to charity, and using the remains for their own enjoyment. Truly, hoarding never brings happiness, and we are deluded if we think it does. Giving always brings happiness, and we are deluded if we think it does not.

Just as a morsel dropped from an elephant's mouth can feed innumerable smaller creatures, a powerful person who becomes a philanthropist can alleviate the pain of countless people. But everyone whether rich or poor can give generously. Offering yourself in service, or simply bestowing the comfort of a kind word or glance, can change the life of a person in despair. Indeed, those who have suffered through their own pains are positioned to be special messengers of solace and consolation.

The sages have said many other things about dana. Two principles are noteworthy. The first is that charity must be offered without any thought that something will be returned in the future. Dana is a selfless offering, and not an exchange or contract. This teaching is sometimes expressed succinctly as "give and forget."

The second principle is that whenever possible dana should not be announced publicly but rendered anonymously and to not garner acclaim. Dana should be given like Mother Nature, who secretly fills the clouds with the water that brings forth abundant food from the earth. This teaching is sometimes distilled into the maxim "give secretly."

Yet even when given freely and secretly, an act of true dana remains engraved in the donor's memory, whose heart receives a lasting stream of joy. This is because our true nature is a reflection of nature itself, but that can only be known when our actions contain a bit of nature's generosity.

20. WORSHIPPING THE LORD / ISHVARA PUJANA

Not everyone has a devotional nature and wants to worship the Lord.[3] But seekers who do encounter a real dilemma. They ask themselves, "How can I worship a Lord who is unknown and invisible?" In trying to answer this question, they might reason: "I am told that worship is a way to express my love, but I have no image or memory of a beloved. To remember someone, there must be an acquaintance in the past, but the Lord is totally unfamiliar to me. Ishvara Pujana means to remember and worship Ishvara in order to know the Lord. How can I love and remember a Lord whom I have never met or seen?"

The mind of a seeker asking questions like this grows exhausted and confused. Imagine them setting out on a pilgrimage to solve this dilemma. Traveling to multiple saints, they humbly inquire, "Have you seen the Lord?" Some of the saints answer affirmatively and gladly provide a description of the Lord's form. But upon comparison, the seeker finds variations and discrepancies. The devotional heart of the seeker wants to believe the Lord exists. Yet another question must be asked, "Are these saints deluded?"

Perhaps an answer can be found in the science of psychology, which says that human beings tend to conceptualize God in their own likeness. This explains why most religions envision the Lord as having a body just like our own. However, the seeker's activated mind wants to carry this point a little further and asks, "How would a buffalo envision the ruler of the cosmos?" The answer seems clear. Naturally, the animal would imagine the Lord is a buffalo.

Joking aside, this dilemma regarding the Lord's form is real and complicated. However, it can be resolved in practice. Here is the most important thing to keep in mind when worshiping the Lord. Although you must

---

[3] Ishvara literally means "the one who possesses the power" and is generally translated as Lord. Ishvara is God in the form of a Supreme Being with whom one can have a personal relationship, in contrast to the impersonal, transcendent, and formless Brahman.

visualize the Lord according to your own conception, have faith and pray in this way. "My intelligence is limited. I am unable to accurately imagine your form in my mind, or hold it clearly in my memory. Yet my heart tells me that you exist in some form or another. Lord, I crave to have your darshan (audience and glimpse) but can only do so with your grace."

For those with an intellectual temperament, the scriptures of Sanatana Dharma clarify the nature of God. A conceptual structure is expounded which elaborately explains how everything emanates from the formless Brahman. It is from this Brahman that the Supreme Spirit of Ishvara emerges, who is considered the Almighty Lord of the universe. Next are the three primary deities that create (Brahma), sustain (Vishnu), and transform (Shiva) the macrocosm. Then comes all of the natural forces, which are seen as divine energies symbolized by various gods and goddesses. Last are the elements from which material existence takes shape. In this way, Sanatana Dharma presents a description of a God who is both with form and without form. A seeker can choose to worship any of these divine expressions. In the form of Ishvara, God is the Lord whose divine will governs this universe.

The sages of old did not speculate to arrive at a conception of God. Instead, they were truth seekers and devotees who sought yoga – union with Truth or God—through prayer, religious rites, pranayama, meditation, self-inquiry, and other techniques. Sanatana Dharma resulted from their deep interior contemplation. A seeker cannot begin Ishvara Pujana until a desire to know and unite with the Lord arises within them. When this occurs, a seeker's best bet is to study trustworthy scriptures until a form of the Lord is found that appeals to their mind and heart. Conceiving an image of that deity, they should inject their feelings into its form and devotionally worship it with a steady mind. As the seeker's mind and heart is purified, their love for the Lord will grow.

Now I will tell you one last thing, which is very important. When a child is born, the parents select a name it will be known by. Likewise, when love for the Lord is born in a seeker's heart, the seeker may choose the name he wants to give to the Lord. This name can be applied to the Lord whether the seeker's conception is with or without form. It is by the use of this chosen name that the Lord can be constantly remembered. That is why in India the name is likened to a footpath that a seeker can walk all the way to the Lord's holy presence.

21. LISTENING TO THE DOCTRINES / SIDDHANTA SRAVANA

A person desiring to learn a particular subject goes to university and studies the best literature in that field. That same principle applies to anyone wanting to attain mastery in yoga. The physical sciences are prospering in the modern age, but their devotion to a strict materialism is limiting because it ignores a portion of the truth. Yoga science as articulated by its ancient scriptures offers a needed complement.

The sublime secrets of the scriptures cannot be comprehended merely by reading them. Reading is only a first step through which you gain a basic familiarity. After that, an effort should be made to receive the scriptures directly from the mouth of a masterful teacher. This is why the niyama is called "listening to the doctrines." In India, it is recognized that the scriptures have multiple layers of meaning. Moreover, it's known that the deepest meanings have been purposefully concealed because they are only useful when received by a student ready to take in that lesson. This is why the need for a teacher is accepted.

The scriptures provide the principles needed to inform a particular approach to yoga practice. After that knowledge is acquired, you can begin to conduct your own experiments. Gradually, you will understand the scriptural knowledge you gained better and better. It is when your practice matures that you really need the scriptures. It is very difficult to reach to the highest without their help.

My guidance is for a yoga student to begin by studying the Ramayana, Mahabharat, and Shrimad Bhagavatam. These great stories (cultural epics) contain innumerable facts that convey the essence of the dharmic culture that gave birth to yoga. In India, children hear these stories continually during their childhood. After that, the Bhagavad Gita should be studied. The Gita is considered foremost among the scriptures because all the scientific and spiritual principles of yoga are distilled into its eighteen dramatic chapters. The great sage Vyasa says that Lord Krishna milked all the cows of the Vedas and Upanishads and churned it into the nectar-like butter of the Gita.

Even though the Bhagavad Gita reveals the highest yogic knowledge, a student may want to also study the Yoga Sutra and Hatha Yoga Pradipika. The specialty of these scriptures is their terseness. Only the ultimate questions and techniques to answer them are considered in compact aphorisms. There is no storyline or other discussion. These scriptures cannot be read like books. A short section is studied intently with a steady mind, after which one goes into contemplation.

A dedicated yogi must constantly strike a balance between the continual practice of yogic techniques and study of the scriptures. The secrets of scriptures are revealed only by this combined practice. Comparing your spiritual experiences with scriptural doctrine, your mind will become less restless, more discriminating, and increasingly established in higher knowledge. At the holy moment when your own experience matches a scriptural statement, your joy will be boundless.

22. HUMILITY / HRI

Today I will discuss the niyama known as hri or humility. History shows us that moral and ethical codes are inherent to civilization. Complex societies do not arise without such codes, and the values of psychology and religion permeate them. While developed by people, there is also something divine in them that points in the direction of our higher nature. It is important to know that these codes exist not only to promote the social order, but also to develop the character of individuals.

When a person of good character transgresses the boundaries of these codes a sense of remorse arises in their heart and mind. This type of conscience does not exist in everyone. Such agitation only arises in the heart of one who accepts that these behavioral norms are necessary and feels bound to follow them to foster the welfare of all. This is a healthy sign of their good intentions and capacity for humility.

Others see these moral and ethical codes differently. They deem them superficial means to foster the social order that do not apply to them. Such individuals consider these norms as etiquette or a pretense of good manners meant only to be displayed publicly. If their desires are thwarted by such rules and principles, they get angry and seek out strategies to satisfy them anyway. These are unhealthy signs of their selfish intentions and capacity for hypocrisy.

One who does not consider others to be their equal cannot advance very far spiritually. Without this degree of humility, it is difficult to receive new knowledge from outside of our egotistical system. An empty cup must bow before a pitcher. A cup that holds itself above any vessels capable of filling it will remain empty. All the spiritual traditions say this. Arrogance must be recognized as an impenetrable barrier on the path to truth. This is why Christ taught, "Blessed are the meek."

Humility cannot be gauged by whether transgressions do or do not occur. In fact, transgressions of these codes inevitably occur even in the life of a vigilant individual. A truth seeker should expect to face dilemmas so complex and stressful that steadiness abandons them and knowingly or unknowingly these transgressions happen. It is not coincidence that this is Arjuna's fate in the Bhagavad Gita. Humility can only be assessed by whether a genuine sense of regret and remorse arises in their heart and mind. And whether they remain honest, sincere in their desire to make amends, and accepting of the rightful bonds established by their society. A humble individual sees clearly that these are not binding limits but the true means to happiness and freedom.

Next to the vastness of truth, a human being is the size of an atom. It is only by truth's greatness that it may choose to descend to the human level. A seeker should never try to cut truth down to size. Instead, they should humbly accept the need to alter themselves. Why? Not to practice the niyama of humility, but because this is the only way to move from insignificance to true greatness, and it fits within the natural laws of development.

23. MANTRA RECITATION / JAPA

In India, the practice of mantra recitation is well established. Countless individuals have experienced the power of a mantra to act as an antidote to their complaints and sufferings. Children grow up hearing the traditional yogic mantras. In all of society, few other practices command such conviction and faith, all of which help the mantra bestow its benefits.

Mantra yoga is a complete path through which an aspirant can attain all four aims of life. The niyama of mantra recitation or japa is the first phase of this path that can be practiced by everyone. Like every other niyama, it is a tool to enhance our positive qualities and help restrain us when we might behave negatively. But when the practice of japa is properly understood, mantra's power to accomplish these things is unparalleled.

First you must establish your practice in the meditation room. Everyone's life is full of problems. Whatever difficulties are troubling you, whatever circumstances are creating fear or disturbance, just drop your thoughts about these things and start your japa (mantra recitation). Merely pronouncing the words is not enough. You must engage all of your attention in the mantra and attune to its sound and meaning. Whatever your particular pain or unhappiness may be, offer it into the stream of japa, and momentarily be free from all worries and concerns.

Our memory is a sea of past incidents. When you sit for japa, the gates to this sea are opened. What psychologists call "free association" brings up past incidents one after another, and the mind may also travel into the future. Distractions of all sorts will continually arise in the mind. Return your attention again and again to the mantra – this is how distraction is overcome and the mind is purified.

Once the practice is understood, it can be engaged outside of the meditation room in life. Imagine you are driving along and find yourself worrying. Noticing that, remain relaxed and begin to mentally chant your mantra. If the mind continues to brood over unhelpful thoughts, increase the speed of your japa slightly. Shifting your attention in this way, anxiety and depression can be avoided.

Done regularly, a mantra becomes so embedded in the mind that once japa is started no outside thought forms can penetrate the recitation. In olden days, this was described as entering a temple and locking the doors so no worries can come in behind you. In our times, it might be likened to flipping on a light switch that illumines the mind and casts out the shadows of inner darkness. But mantra is not only a remedy for problems. If done with one-pointed concentration, you will derive great joy from it. This joy of mantra has the power to change every cell of your body and synapse of your mind.

Buddhism, Judaism, Christianity, Islam and some schools of psychology have a tradition of mantra (or affirmation) repetition. At this stage of niyama in which mental weaknesses are being removed and the ability to focus and direct the mind is being strengthened, any mantra can be used. For those wanting to practice mantra yoga, it is important to receive a divinely-inspired mantra from a guru who became realized through this approach and is thus fit to initiate and instruct you in its practice.

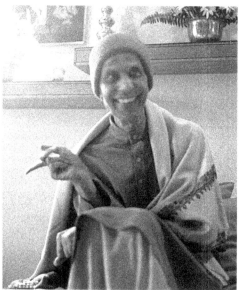
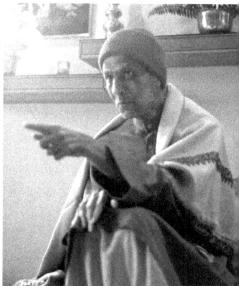

Swami Kripalu telling a story near the end of his life as photographed by Deborah Dorn.

APPENDIX 2

TEACHING STORIES

Modern life is such that everyone is constantly busy with external work. As a teacher, I've come to see that listening to lectures occurs to busy people like eating gruel. They much prefer the ambrosia of a story. Where sermons fall flat and are not even retained by those who hear them, a story rouses attention and exits the lecture hall to spread everywhere. That is why I dress up my explanations of yoga in the garb of stories.

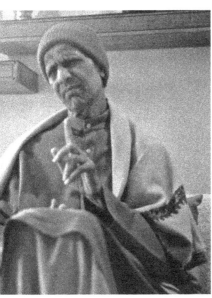

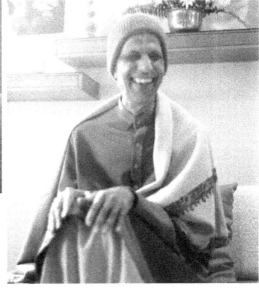

Swami Kripalu was at heart a storyteller, an activity he loved but also reflects a method of instruction native to the yoga tradition. Many of the tales he told come from the Puranas, a word that means "old stories" and refers to a distinct genre of literature that preserves the legends and lore of traditional India. Among literary scholars, the Puranas are famed for their intricate layering of symbolic meaning. A single story may teach an obvious moral lesson, show how a character's values or chosen actions play out over time, and be interpretable on an entirely different level to reveal a profound mystical truth. Other stories he told are contemporary, including anecdotes from his life, and a number of tradition-like stories he apparently made up.

It is fitting that he packaged his instruction on how to hear—or read—these stories in a parable. The Christian metaphor of a large animal passing through the eye of a needle stands out and suggests he may have adapted an older Indian story to get his message across to a Western audience:

Students and disciples have a habit of always bowing and saying yes to their teachers. In India, this is considered good manners and a way of showing respect. Once there was a Jain acharya (masterful teacher) who saw this trait being displayed in a meeting hall that he was about to address. This acharya taught in the traditional way by telling stories. He knew this habit had to be addressed before he could effectively teach the audience anything. Suddenly the acharya had an idea, and acting on it he began his lecture.

"Jain brothers and sisters, are you willing to listen to me tonight?" In one voice, all the people gathered answered, "Ji," which means "Yes." He continued, "Once there was a great elephant," to which everyone again replied, "Yes." "While out walking and looking at the ground, this elephant's sharp vision spotted a sewing needle standing up on its point." Again, the group said in unison, "Yes." "This elephant became very curious about the hole in that needle. Lowering his head, his focus was such that his body passed through the eye of the needle." The crowd did not miss a beat—"Yes." "But the very end of the elephant's tail got caught in the hole and would not pass through," To which yet again, the assemblage said, "Yes."

Only now could the acharya begin his real teaching. "Brother and sister truth seekers. Why are you saying "yes" to all this nonsense? Everyone knows an elephant cannot go through the eye of a needle. On top of that, I told you the elephant's massive body went through but then his skinny tail got caught. Please ask yourself: What is the good of this unthinking yes that I am saying to everything? Most certainly, stories are mysterious. They may be metaphorical and have hidden symbolism. But in order to have meaning their message must somehow be pointing us toward truth. Respectfully I say, you must listen and think more deeply to understand the stories I have to tell from the Jain dharma.

The hall fell suddenly silent. Having broken their habit of saying yes to everything, the acharya could now continue his instruction with an audience able to thoughtfully receive his words.

Here is a complete list of the teaching stories told or referenced in this book along with the page number where they appear. Those stories appended here are ones that did not appear earlier in the book. Each is briefly introduced, told in SK's words, and followed by a commentary. Readers wanting to continue their study of these teaching stories are directed to the works of past ashram resident and author, John Mundhal.[1]

Don't Discount Your Self 48
The Saint and the Scorpion 82
The Ten Thousand Rupee Teaching 172
The Tax Collector and the Mahatma 284
The Farmer's Vow 286
The Sculptor and His Son 289
The Life of Lord Buddha 293
Mantra Yoga and Anahat Nada 302
The Women and Their Dearest Treasure 305
The Marriage of Divarka and Kalpalata 308
The Nature of a Yogi 311

---

[1] *From the Heart of the Lotus: The Teaching Stories of Swami Kripalu*, compiled and edited by John Mundahl (Monkfish, 2008).

THE TAX COLLECTOR AND THE MAHATMA

Swami Kripalu spent over a decade as an itinerant spiritual teacher. At first, he traveled on foot from village to village in the Narmada River district. As his reputation spread, he became a celebrated public figure and spoke at locations throughout the Indian state of Gujarat. This story has no apparent author, which is a good clue that it is original to SK. While serving in a role much like that of the Mahatma depicted in this story, it's likely he encountered numerous individuals whose characters he blended together to create the overly self-important Tax Collector.

There once was a Tax Collector who had grown haughty from all the flattery heaped upon him by rich people seeking to lower their tax bills. One day an influential business man came to his office and ended their meeting by saying, "Good sir, there is a Mahatma visiting the city and giving audience to all the people. Last night, I attended his lecture and was greatly inspired. My heart would like you to receive his teachings too." The Tax Collector replied, "I've heard of this Mahatma and would like to meet him, but only if it's possible for the two of us to speak personally." Pleased with this positive response, the business man continued, "After the Mahatma was done speaking last night, I introduced myself to his top student and made a gift to support their work. Come a little before seven o'clock tonight, and I'll make all the arrangements."

When the Tax Collector arrived, he was pleased to find the Mahatma sitting alone in the front of a large room. Making his way forward, the Tax Collector passed through a group of students and city elders gathered in the back discussing how to manage the crowd that would soon arrive. The Mahatma noticed right away that the Tax Collector was some special person, as all the city elders moved aside and saluted him.

Greeting the Mahatma, the Tax Collector bowed his head slightly and said, "Mahatmaji, I am happy to be at your feet. I have read many scriptures and thought deeply about religion. I've come early to meet with you alone, and not with all the common people, so you can give me a teaching suitable to me." The Mahatma could see the Tax Collector was filled with pride. Yet he spoke lovingly and with great peace, saying just a single word: "Dharma."

The Tax Collector waited for the Mahatma to continue. Thirty seconds passed in silence before the Tax Collector asked a second question: "What exactly do you mean?" The Mahatma responded: "Always do right. Whenever possible, avoid doing wrong. Regard others as your own self and work to meet their needs. Be grateful to God, who has provided us this world in which to live. All these are dharma." His face twisting into a sneer, the Tax Collector's response was immediate. "I already know all that. Tell me something more advanced than this ordinary teaching."

The Mahatma looked directly into the Tax Collector's eyes and again uttered a single word, this time in a voice audible all the way in the back of the room, "Fool." At this the Tax Collector's anger boiled over. "I'm an important city official. In front of all these people, you have insulted me!"

Once again, the Mahatma spoke lovingly and with great peace, "Pardon me if you felt insulted. All I did was say the word fool. It is clear to me that you know its meaning because of the effect it had on you. However, when I said the word dharma, there was no change in you at all. As a spiritual teacher, I have to question whether you truly know its meaning."

In that moment, the Tax Collector realized that this Mahatma was speaking the truth to him. Humbled, his eyes looked downward and he fell silent. The Mahatma was silent too, but there was no break in his presence or peacefulness. A minute passed during which the Tax Collector experienced a genuine change of heart. Lifting his eyes to meet the Mahatma's loving gaze, the Tax Collector said, "You are right. I am just a beginning student. If it is acceptable to you, I will now take a seat for your public discourse."

It's easy for anyone whose interest in yoga has been kindled to imagine the only important task before them is to learn its advanced practices aimed at spiritual awakening. This story counters that naïve notion by affirming that yoga will only bear fruit when done by a person willing to persevere in the basic lifestyle practices and cultivate a humble and virtuous character.

THE FARMER'S VOW

Some of the stories told by Swami Kripalu seem like sheer tomfoolery. A casual listener laughs and afterward goes on, assuming his only purpose was inserting a little comic relief into an otherwise dry lecture. But a student who realizes that his wit was undergirded by a steely intentionality listens harder to discern the story's deeper significance. This humorous story has a message for both beginning and advancing yoga practitioners.

> *Once a true saint arrived in a small town. Within a few days, the people recognized his divine qualities and the elders of the community asked him, "Please let us drink the nectar of your teachings." The saint agreed and the town's inhabitants gathered for a series of discourses. A month passed and during that time the saint inspired many to perform spiritual practices. As a result, the town became peaceful and everyone treated each other with special respect. When the time came for the saint to depart, the people were sad, but he comforted them by announcing a farewell discourse.*
>
> *That night there was a farmer in the crowd who had come into town a few times to hear the saint speak. He wasn't interested in religion or spiritual growth, yet the saint had inspired him too. When the discourse was over the farmer approached the saint. "Mahatma, I am not interested in God or yoga. I'm always busy working my fields. I'm unable to undertake a difficult practice. What should I do?"*
>
> *The saint respected the farmer's honesty and replied with love. "Take a vow you find easy. By observing it, your will power will increase, your life will become disciplined, and you will become able to succeed at whatever you wish." The farmer was in unfamiliar territory. As a result, his mind grew agitated causing him to stammer out, "But I can't decide what vow to make. Please give me a simple discipline to practice."*
>
> *"Very well," the saint said. "For six months, eat your evening meal only after doing some act." The farmer calmed down. "That's simple enough," he said. "Will any act do?" "Yes, what you do is not important," the saint explained. "Your determination to observe the vow is what's vital. This is only a preliminary practice, but if*

undertaken it will produce a definite result." After saying this, the saint blessed the farmer, who left inspired to make a vow.

Once the farmer got home, he thought things over. "Maybe I could go to the temple before I eat? But I'm always hungry after working all day. The Shiva temple is too far. The Krishna temple is nearby, but it's not always open. If I make a vow that I can't easily fulfill, then I cannot eat dinner even if I'm starving. I'd better be careful about this."

Just then the farmer looked up and saw his neighbor's old donkey standing in the pasture between their houses. His neighbor was a potter and never used the donkey. Every morning, when the farmer set out for his fields, the donkey could be seen standing there looking in his direction. When the farmer returned in the evening, the stubborn animal would be standing in the same exact spot. "This is a great idea," the farmer thought. "For the next six months, I will only eat my dinner after seeing the donkey's face."

Five months passed and each day the farmer was able to wash up and glance at the donkey to see his face before eating, so he kept his vow without any problem. As the rainy season approached the farmer's workload increased, but he was still able to get back from his fields with enough light in the sky to see the donkey. Then one evening, after an especially hard day, the farmer arrived home famished. Sitting down at his table, the donkey was not there. His thwarted hunger quickly turned to anger. He got mad at the saint for inspiring him to take a vow. He got mad at himself for foolishly making it. He got mad at his neighbor, and the stubborn old donkey too. "What good is this vow?" he said, "I am going to give it up." After feeling this flood of anger, his determination returned. "All my life, I've never committed myself to anything other than farm work," he said to himself. "This is my first chance to honor a spiritual commitment, and it isn't right for me to break it."

Driven by hunger, he walked quickly to his neighbor's house. Only his son was home, and the farmer asked, "Where has your father gone with his donkey?" The boy answered, "He and my mother are behind the house digging sand from the hillside." The farmer headed toward them, and in a short time he could see them on the hill, but the donkey had his backside to him. Since he had vowed to look at the donkey's face, he couldn't return after only seeing the donkey's tail, so he continued to walk until he came quite close.

Unbeknownst to the farmer, something extraordinary was happening to the potter and his wife. While digging sand to make clay, they had found a chest full of gold jewelry. After hugging each other in ecstasy, they got the donkey to help them haul the heavy chest to the house. Too jubilant to be watchful, they hadn't noticed the farmer's approach.

After seeing the donkey's face, the farmer turned and began walking away. The potter concluded that the farmer had seen the treasure and was going to tell the authorities. "We must convince our neighbor not to tell," the farmer said to his wife. "The government will take the whole fortune!" She immediately agreed.

"Good neighbor," the potter yelled. "Wait a minute." The farmer glanced back, but he was lost in thought about his vow and hunger. So he said, "Yes, I've seen it," meaning the donkey's face. The potter misunderstood and was now certain the farmer had seen the treasure. "Dear neighbor," the potter said in a sweet voice. "We know you've seen the treasure chest we dug up. But if you report this to the authorities none of us will benefit. It would be best to keep quiet and divide the treasure between us."

The farmer had no idea what the potter was talking about, but he wisely remained silent. Only after he walked back to where the potter and his wife were standing did he see the hole in the ground and the open chest. Understanding the situation, he consented to his neighbor's proposal, convinced that his vow had brought him this boon. Bundling his share of the treasure in his coat, the farmer headed home. That night he ate his evening meal peacefully with a contented mind. Seeing how the saint's prediction that observing a vow would produce a definite result had come true, his faith in the power of practice grew strong.

After hearing this story, you may ask, "If I observe spiritual disciplines, will I also discover treasure?" Yes, I can say that if you practice with determination, you will definitely find treasure, buried not in the earth, but in the depths of your own heart and soul.

While the story ends at the farmer's dinner table, it's easy to imagine its epilogue. Inspired by the outcome of his vow, the farmer continues on the spiritual path with great faith. Having tasted the benefits of performing a "preliminary practice," he experiments with a more-primary practice like mantra meditation. Freed from the need to perform dawn-to-dusk manual labor, he is able to persevere in it and make real spiritual progress. This is SK's message to beginning students, whom he trusted would emerge from an initial period of practice inspired to delve more deeply into yoga.

His message to seasoned students is harder to discern. Anyone advancing to the later stages of yoga will have gained the knowledge needed to inform a systematic yoga practice. When it's clearly understood that yoga is a way to methodically remove tensions and blocks from every layer and level of our being so the light and love of an all-pervading consciousness can shine forth unobstructed, one's initial efforts at practice will appear haphazard and almost comical.

THE SCULPTOR AND HIS SON

Swami Kripalu lost his father at age seven. In many ways, this traumatic event and its cascade of consequences defined his early life. At age nineteen, he encountered a renunciate sadhu (holy man) who accepted him as a spiritual son. For a year-and-a-quarter, they lived together in the sadhu's Bombay ashram, which enabled the sadhu to school SK in the principles of yoga. An eager and gifted student, he was also opinionated and at times obstinate. Near the end of his tutelage, the patient sadhu believed in his student enough to initiate him into yoga's deeper teachings and practices. In many ways, the events of this year-and-a-quarter would define his later life. Given his history, it is easy to understand why in this story he depicts the ideal guru/disciple relationship as one of a caring father and his talented, highly-motivated, and headstrong son.

> *Once there was a well-known sculptor named Ratneshvar who had a son named Devarshi. From an early age, Devarshi wanted to follow in the footsteps of his father. Accepting this as his son's chosen aim in life, Ratneshvar guided his development. Devarshi was*

a keen student and mastered the basic techniques of sculpting in childhood. During his teenage years, his father was able to instruct him in many advanced techniques. By the age of twenty, Devarshi's work was being recognized all over India.

Whenever Devarshi's work received acclaim, he would run to his father. "This famous person has praised my sculpture!" Ratneshvar was a true artist, and as skilled at teaching as he was at sculpting. He would listen affectionately and then say, "Yes, I also like this work of yours. But artistic excellence only develops gradually. To understand the secrets of sculpture, you must practice for many years. Every great young artist of the past felt just as you do now. As they matured and went deeper into their work, they realized that only by creating many pieces can an artist embody the subtlety of his art."

Devarshi didn't like this speech. One day he told his father, "You never rate my pieces as highly as the gallery critics. You are withholding your true opinion from me." Ratneshwar understood his son's feelings. He knew the value of encouragement. Yet he also understood that flattery can stunt the development of an artist by clouding his creative faculty and causing him to stop growing. He evaluated Devarshi's works as a fellow sculptor and not as an art critic. First, he praised all its good features, and then he explored its flaws. He believed a true artist was one who welcomed constructive criticism. He explained, "The critics who praise your work are lovers of sculpture. They see you as a budding artist in need of inspiration through praise. I am a sculptor myself, and much more familiar with you and your work. I give you my complete and honest assessment to help you improve." Despite this explanation, Devarshi still felt hurt, and disagreements of this type kept occurring between them.

Devarshi continued to work hard and always placed new pieces in his father's hands, asking for his opinion. Sensitive to Devarshi's feelings, Ratneshwar deliberately avoided pointing out any faults. Knowing that his son still needed guidance, he found a way to provide it indirectly. Praising Devarshi's piece, he would compare it to that of another sculptor striving to overcome similar deficits. Devarshi was familiar with the work of these artists and quick to recognize his own shortcomings in their pieces. Often, he spotted the flaw immediately and exclaimed, "Father, I made the same mistake in the sculpture I just created." This is the method Ratneshwar used to keep his son inspired and growing.

One day a sculpture of Devarshi's won first prize in an exhibition. The critics called it "an extraordinary work of art" and said that Devarshi was destined to become one of the top sculptors in the country. When his father didn't fully agree, Devarshi was frustrated. He was convinced that his father was stingily holding back his praise. Angry and hurt, he devised a plan to force his father to reveal his true opinion.

Devarshi began a new piece. As he worked in secret, he initiated conversations with his father on the finest nuances of sculpture, which he then employed in his project. Ratneshwar was delighted to witness his son's sharp mind. With joy and affection, he conveyed all his remaining knowledge to his son. Ratneshwar's true wish was for Devarshi to surpass him in his artistry and achievements. When his secret sculpture was finished, Devarshi traveled to the site of an ancient shrine and current archeological dig. Rubbing his new piece in the dirt, he buried it where it was sure to be found. Six months later, the newspapers were full of articles on what was described as an ancient piece of sculpture unearthed at the site. Ratneshwar's attention was naturally drawn to these stories. He read the published descriptions of the find with great interest and was intrigued by their beautiful photographs. One morning he told his son, "Devarshi, let us travel to this shrine. We'll see and learn many things there."

Devarshi agreed and upon reaching their destination they entered a throng of people drawn by the recent publicity. Since father and son were well-known sculptors, the organizers welcomed them warmly and assigned a guide to show them the site and its ancient remains. At the end of the day, they were ushered into an empty viewing room and allowed to inspect the unique piece of art that had recently been excavated. The tour guide left for a moment, and father and son stood alone.

Ratneshwar's attention was absorbed by the statue displayed at the center of the room. After examining it carefully, he *exclaimed, "Devarshi, this is the best piece of sculpture I've ever seen, ancient or modern. I see in this work certain concepts that I myself have been trying to express but so far have only been able to imagine. The vision of this unknown sculptor is truly timeless, for instilled in this single piece is a beautiful balance of ancient and contemporary styles, with intimations of future art as well. This is the path along which I'm trying to lead you."*

Devarshi lifted the statue from its pedestal and turned it upside down. On the bottom was his name written in his characteristic lettering. Ratneshwar's eyes filled with tears of joy. "My son," he said. "By not overly praising your pieces, I was trying to prevent you from becoming egotistical. Art is an ocean and the artist a drop. No matter how skilled, an artist always fails to accommodate the ocean of possibilities in the droplet of his lifework. Art can never be produced to earn awards or material gain. Art is creating something beautiful purely for the sake of creation. In the ardent struggle to produce a genuine masterpiece is found divine joy, the artist's true reward."

Devarshi was moved by his father's heartfelt utterance and high ideals. Bowing down, he said, "I am your son by birth. Please bless me that I may become a disciple who embodies your principles in life." Embracing his son, Ratneshwar said, "You already have my blessing. Through genuine artistry, may you become the greatest sculptor in all of India."

India in the era of the Puranas was culturally rich in all of the arts including sculpture. It's likely that Swami Kripalu adapted a traditional tale to produce this more-contemporary teaching story. Many themes can be spotted in its careful reading. Perhaps the most important is the need for a continual evolution of the artist, and refinement of their skills, through lifelong practice. As teacher and student, Devarshi and his father must navigate a steadily shifting balance of instruction and autonomy.

The events leading to Devarshi's "graduation" are especially interesting. One easy-to-miss element is the significance of the signature borne by his buried sculpture. An artist's true work is the person they become via the artistic process. It's also noteworthy that Devarshi's crowning art piece is indistinguishable from the works of the great artists of India's past. This suggests that any authentic Self-realization should correspond to the standards set by the original yoga masters in their texts and—as Swami Kripalu adds—simultaneously reflect our current evolutionary potential.

Only at the end of his tutelage does Devarshi vocally accept his father as his guru. This mirrors the arc of SK's relationship with his own teacher. SK advised yoga aspirants against taking initiation from gurus whom they did not know well from close and personal experience.

THE LIFE OF LORD BUDDHA

Yoga and Buddhism are both rooted in the ancient Vedic culture. While sharing many beliefs and doctrines, they are independent systems of thought. On a few key issues, they take opposing philosophical positions that adherents have hotly debated for centuries. While alert to these differences in view, Swami Kripalu chose to emphasize their essential similarity. Each advocates a systematic path of yogic practice that leads to depth meditation and spiritual awakening. SK felt that Buddha's life story epitomizes the path of yoga and had no reservations placing it front and center in the education of his western students.

> *In the time of Lord Buddha, his personality and charisma were such that anyone in India hearing his name would lower their head in respect and awe. The greatness of such a master cannot be conveyed in words, but today I will tell you his story because it expresses how the truth can be found.*
>
> *Buddha was born in the foothills of the Himalayas in the region now known as Nepal. His father was a king who loved his subjects. Celebration broke out upon the queen's birth of a son, as the good king finally had a successor. The child was given the name Siddhartha, which means "one who will fulfill all four aims of life." The astrologers gathered in the palace and declared that prince Siddhartha was destined for greatness. He would either be the greatest of rulers or the greatest of saints. The royal family was concerned by this prophesy. Their region was inhabited by many sramanas (spiritual strivers) and yogis who carried out their practices*

in the nearby mountains. Now that they had a son, it distressed them to think that one day he might renounce the world to become a saint.

The king called together his ministers to help him determine how to proceed. They decided to make all efforts to shield the prince from ever being exposed to even the slightest pain or suffering. Why did the king and ministers think this way? They knew that anyone who becomes a spiritual master must first confront the truth of human suffering. The astrologers kept silent when this plan was announced, as they knew that nobody can interfere with another's destiny.

Even from an early age there was something unusual about prince Siddhartha. He participated in the palace training given all members of the ruling class, but he stood out as the most intelligent of the boys. He always proved victorious in the competitions held to test their skill in handling the weapons of war. He was also heartfelt, treating the people and animals that lived on the palace grounds with great love.

Hearing of these qualities, the people of the city were eager to see the young prince. Arrangements were made for him to make a procession through the city. A fixed route was set. Anyone whose appearance might disturb his happiness was ordered not to attend, and many other precautions were taken. The morning of the procession arrived and everywhere people lined the roads. As the prince passed, girls and young women came close to offer him flowers. Dignitaries waved from the verandas of their palatial homes. The entire city was jubilant and other special events were held so the prince could see the citizens who would one day be his subjects.

When prince Siddhartha turned fifteen, a second procession was organized to mark his entry into adulthood. The prince was seated on a big elephant at its head. Everything was going as planned when he suddenly directed the elephant handler, "Don't go that way – go this way." The way the prince was pointing was off the fixed route. The handler was confused but had to follow the order of the royal prince, who was now a man. All the people in charge of the procession were following behind. Their hearts started beating heavily. Nobody could imagine what would happen next.

As soon as they left the fixed route, the prince saw an elderly man for the first time in his life. The old man was trying to get out of the way of the elephant. Placing his stick on the ground, he started walking in the other direction, but his legs would not move quickly. Under the effort, his whole body started shaking. The prince ordered his handler, "Let the elephant sit." With slow steps the prince approached the old man, whose sunken eyes were surrounded by wrinkled skin. His hair was white and his cheeks were hollow. Leaning on his stick, the old man smiled at the prince, who could see that many of the man's teeth were missing. One of the ministers appeared and the prince asked him, "What is this?" The minister answered, "My dear prince, this is old age. When a child is born, it grows up and gradually becomes old." The prince was incredulous, "Does everyone go through this?" The minister was forced to answer "yes" as he ushered the prince back to his seat on the elephant.

The procession moved on, but soon the prince saw a man lying by the roadside with open sores and pus oozing from his body. Once again, he debarked from his elephant and the minister had to explain. "My dear prince, this man is suffering from disease. Whenever a disturbance arises in the body, it causes one of many different kinds of diseases. Everyone sooner or later becomes the victim of one of these diseases." Prince Siddhartha was revolted by the woeful condition of the diseased man, and the minister escorted him back onto the elephant with great difficulty.

The procession continued and was turning a corner to return to its fixed route when the prince's eyes fell upon the body of a man being carried to the cremation ground. Once again, he got off his elephant, and the minister was quickly at his side. Seeing the lifeless man strapped to the carrier, the prince asked, "Why doesn't this man move? Is he sleeping?" The minister replied, "My lord, this man is dead. No longer will he move, or talk, or be able to do anything. His body will be burned."

The prince's mind was straining to understand everything he had seen. He inquired of the minister, "This world has existed for countless ages. Hasn't anyone tried to find a solution to this problem of old age, disease, and death?" Such questions do not come from a worldly ruler; these are the questions of a yogi. The minister was forced to admit, "This earth is very old and innumerable people have been born on it, but all of them have died. This body of ours grows old. Eventually it is overtaken by disease and death. This cycle cannot be prevented."

The procession wended its way back to the palace, but prince Siddhartha was unable to see anything else. When the king and queen came to receive him, they could tell right away he was greatly disturbed. They tried to console their son, but from that day forward the consciousness of the prince was changed. Deeply etched in his mind was the memory of the old man, the diseased man, and the corpse. He tried to overcome this state and bring joy to his parents by smiling when conducting his public duties, but palace life no longer held any appeal. Whenever he entered his private chambers, his thoughts would become serious. His mind had turned to his real mission in life, which was to discover a way to counteract suffering and share it with the world.

A year passed and the royal family decided the prince should be married to change the direction of his mind. A festival was arranged and the best of princesses invited. Each young woman was given time to demonstrate her arts and specialties with awards given to the top finishers. The festival was to be presided over by the prince, who would select the winners and hand out the prizes. All the princesses participated, as many were eager to marry the handsome Siddhartha.

A princess named Yasodhara was one of the top finishers. She was beautiful, but also intelligent, and closely observed the mental condition of the prince. When each of the award winners were called to meet with the prince alone, Yasodhara knew that she must talk to him. Standing before him, the prince was surprised when she asked, "What is the cause of your worry?" Prince Siddhartha answered candidly, "You are young and beautiful, but both of us will grow old and die. What good is it to marry?" Yasodhara carefully listened to the thoughts and feelings of the prince. Then she replied, "My prince, these things are bound to happen. It is true that death will come to me, but this worry cannot prevent me from living now." The prince was taken by Yasodhara's directness and told her that he felt called to find a solution to these problems. She promised him, "Should you choose me as a wife, I will cooperate in your svadharma (life purpose). Whatever you need to do, I will support you." The prince was greatly pleased by this exchange, and they were soon married.

A few years passed and Yasodhara gave birth to a son. Where it had taken a long time for his father to produce an heir to the throne, Siddhartha was able to do so quickly. For a great soul destined to pursue the highest, the preliminary aims of life come easily. But Siddhartha had no desire to rule the kingdom. Having satisfied his last royal obligation, the prince withdrew into the depths of his being. Often at night, he pretended to sleep while making plans to escape the palace.

One full moon night, the prince slipped out of his bed just after midnight. He sat quietly for half an hour, reviewing all his thoughts and plans. Having firmly decided, he stood up and silently walked to where Yasodhara was asleep with their son, Rahula. Observing their innocent faces, he folded his two palms and said in his mind to Yasodhara, "I am leaving you only in search of a solution. You have always pleased and served me. You have never offended me in any way. Still, I am leaving you, but not with a cold heart." Gazing at his son, he had no words. Fearing his heart might grow faint, he turned and quickly walked away.

The gatekeeper was surprised to see the prince outside so late at night and called, "May I know your orders." The prince answered, "Bring my horse." The gatekeeper brought the horse the prince had grown up riding and a second for himself, as it wasn't proper for the prince to travel alone. The prince's horse felt that his master wanted to go far away. After passing through the town, they started moving with such speed that they were almost flying. They rode this way until dawn was breaking when they arrived at a river. The prince dismounted with deep appreciation for his horse's service. He hugged the horse, whose mouth was foaming saliva. The horse laid his head on the shoulder of the prince and died, having fulfilled his duty completely. The significance of this event was not lost to Siddhartha—he too was entering a new life.

The gatekeeper had also come down from his horse. One by one, the prince took off all his clothes and ornaments, keeping just a *single cloth wrapped around his waist. Handing the gatekeeper his princely attire, Siddhartha directed him, "Tell the king and queen that I have left to search for a solution. Give my well wishes to everyone." After saying this, he walked quickly away. The gatekeeper was stunned by the prince's announcement and stood like a statue holding the prince's bundle. By the time he came back to his senses, the prince had entered the river and was beyond his reach.*

Siddhartha was now a monk, and over the next six years he conducted his search. He approached the great yogis of his time and became proficient in the practices they taught. He also read many scriptures. Eventually he left these teachers, but that does not mean he rejected them. He learned many valuable things during this time, but nothing that provided an answer to his problem, so he moved on.

Next Siddhartha took up the path of asceticism. One practice on this path is to take a cup of rice and count the grains. Each day, the amount of rice eaten is reduced by one grain. When you get to a single grain of rice, you fast. Siddhartha did this practice, and after fasting for many days he could barely stand up. Once erect, he soon fell down. Siddhartha knew that if he continued to fast, his emaciated body would die, and his problem would go unsolved. This is why he chose to leave the path of asceticism and take up the middle path of moderation, which was a great discovery.

If there is any root cause for searching to discover truth, it is suffering from the profound pain of finding no answer to your problem. This might be described as hitting a dead end. The special characteristic of a great master is they continue searching for a solution to the human condition, despite being defeated thousands of times, until just one way through it is found. Having reached the end of all established paths, Siddhartha realized that he needed to conduct his own experiments. He took his seat under a great tree, vowing to stay there until he either found a solution or passed on from this life. Entering meditation, he eventually found the truth that dispels all misery and became the awakened one we know as the Buddha.

Buddha remained under the tree until he had distilled his discovery into four principles. First, suffering exists. Second, there is a reason suffering arises. Third, suffering can be removed. His last principle lists the remedies to remove suffering. These four principles of the Buddha are completely in line with Sanatana Dharma. After experiencing this truth, a great master can give happiness to the world. Buddha spent the next forty-five years traveling on foot throughout northern India and sharing these principles with everyone. Rich or poor, high caste or low, man or woman – all were equal in his sight. People came to call his approach Buddha Dharma.

Buddha's life was long and full of miracles. Today I made it short so you could hear how he found the truth. We are ordinary people seeking only happiness. It is not proper to compare ourselves with an extraordinary person like the Buddha. Yet we must also progress along established paths until the time comes to boldly conduct our own experiments. Then we must be willing to stay at our tasks until they are completed or the prana (vital force) leaves our body, for without the courage of this conviction the work of our life will remain unfinished.

It's been said that history yields no better tale than Buddha's life story. It's a saga that's been told and retold in many different versions over the centuries. Rather than a biography, the relatively small number of facts that scholars can confirm about Siddhartha Gautama's life have become the skeleton of a great myth meant to convey the profound truth of what's possible for individuals to experience and achieve through their own efforts.

Swami Kripalu did not spoon-feed his students, and this relatively brief recounting of Buddha's life was not intended to be a definitive teaching. It was meant to point a student in the direction of further study. Knowing this, any attempt on my part to decipher this epic story in a short commentary would be a disservice to the reader. Many books are available that furnish a full account. My favorite is *The Buddha: His Life Retold* by Robert Allen Mitchell, which preserves the traditional symbolism and provides a sampling of Buddha's most important discourses, both of which imbue the story with transformative power. A discerning student will balance that mythic perspective with a more historical account.

There is an event in Buddha's life that I want to highlight. It came to my attention in an offhand comment made by SK near the end of his talk: *After his awakening, Lord Buddha came back to the kingdom. In their first meeting, Yasodhara asked her husband a very interesting question, one that even the Buddha had trouble answering.*

In the traditional version of the story, Yasodhara is not presented kindly. When her husband returns, eight years after leaving her in the dark of night, and two years after his enlightenment, she is tearful and bitterly angry. In some depictions, her womanly emotions get the better of her, and she refuses to see him. Others provide a mirror image view in which she is the model Indian wife who falls in devotion at her husband's feet. Neither of these grant the character of Yasodhara much depth, or explain SK's comment. But then I came upon this alternative ending to their love story:

> When princess Yasodhara realized that her husband had left to live as a monk, she remained true to her promise to support his quest. While residing in the court, she led a simple life. Still beautiful and a member of the royal family, several princes sought her hand, but she rejected their proposals. For the first six years of his absence, Yasodhara followed the news of her husband's actions closely. Hearing of his enlightenment, she hoped for his return. Anticipation turned to anger and resentment in the two long years when it appeared he had forsaken his family entirely. When word came that the Buddha had arrived in the kingdom, Yasodhara did not go to see her former husband. Instead, she asked her son Rahula to go to his father to confirm his inheritance. Inwardly she thought, "Surely, if I mean anything to him, he will come to me of his own accord."
>
> After greeting his father the king, Buddha came to Yasodhara. He wanted to express his gratitude for her support, and to give to her something of what had happened to him. That much he owed to her. He found Yasodhara not dressed in the costly finery befitting her royal station, but in the simple yellow robes of a nun. Her face, no longer adorned by cosmetic artifice, seemed young and guileless.
>
> Yasodhara lifted her head to look at him through a veil of grief and tears. Immediately, she was struck by his presence. She

thought to herself, "This is not the same man I used to know. He has changed tremendously. No, he is not the same man at all." Looking more closely, she could see that an aura of luminosity surrounded him. She thought, "This is something I have never seen before – a man truly at peace." In these brief moments, Yasodhara's anger departed, and the rage she'd long felt subsided.

Purged of these feelings, Yasodhara regained her composure. Meeting his gaze, she spoke. "Just tell me one thing," she said. "Whatever it is that you have attained in the forest, and I can see that you have attained it, was it not possible for you to attain it here, in this house?"

Now it was the Buddha who had to gaze at the earth. He had never before considered this question. Several moments passed with him staring downward before he could lift his head to answer, "No, I did not have to leave. It could have been attained here in this house." Another silence passed before he completed his response, "But I did not know that then."

Yashoda was satisfied by his answer.

I was intrigued by Swami Kripalu's reference to this non-traditional rendition of the myth, which speaks directly to the householder and renunciate paths, and tried to track down its origin. It appears to spring from a Bengali poem by Rabindranath Tagore, a towering cultural figure who received the Nobel Prize for literature in 1913. Tagore remained a prominent artist and social reformer until his death in 1941. As a working playwright and self-described *lover of literature*, SK would have been aware of Tagore's work. He must have deemed Tagore's questioning of the renunciation ethic worthy enough to include this pointer in his talk.

History provides a generally accepted fact-based ending to Yashoda's story. Their son, Rahula, followed his father into the monastic community shortly after Buddha returned to the kingdom. Five years later, Yasodhara was among a sizeable first group of women ordained as bhikkhunis (Buddhist nuns). During her religious life, she was recognized as an arhat – someone who has attained nirvana by following the teachings of the Buddha. She died at age seventy-eight, two years before her former husband.

MANTRA YOGA AND ANAHAT NADA

Swami Kripalu's depiction of spontaneous sounding or anahat nada as a yogic technique able to reveal divine mantras has a close parallel in Pentecostal and charismatic Christianity. The phenomenon of glossolalia, a Greek word that means "speaking in tongues," dates back to the early Christian church. Moved by the Holy Spirit, believers utter sounds and words in a fluid speech-like cadence and rhythm, usually in states of religious passion. Some denominations consider these utterances to reflect a divine language able to convey direct messages from God. Neuroscientists studying glossolalia through the technology of brain scanning have found that subjects display a marked decrease in frontal lobe activity. This could explain the perceived loss of self-control reported by practitioners.

SK's discovery of anahat nada is recounted in chapter 4 of *Dharma Then Moksha*, which places its practice in the larger context of his energetic and spiritual awakening. There are two basic stages of the practice. In the first, spontaneous sounding is done volitionally as a tool to awaken what SK calls the "primal power" and through it the "evolutionary force." In the second stage, the practice matures into anahat nada, in which the sounding is said to be generated automatically by these awakened energies.

This story provides a window on the experience of a novice practitioner ushered swiftly into an advanced stage of practice. While anahat nada is primarily a renunciate practice, SK considered it the origin point for the broad lexicon of yogic mantras traditionally recited by householders, which is the primary reason this teaching story is featured.

> *It is easy to explain the mantra diksha (initiation) given to commence japa sadhana (practice). It is very difficult to explain the sadhana of anahat nada and the (shaktipat) diksa it requires, but let me give you an example.*
>
> *Lauture Massac is a student of mine who was born in France. He came to India with a list of yogis he wanted to meet. After our first meeting, he asked to me to accept him as a disciple. I answered: "First you must go and meet all these other yogis."*
>
> *After completing this undertaking, Mr. Massac returned and*

offered himself to me saying, "I have accepted you alone as my guru. Please give me training in yoga. I am a sincere seeker. I left my country, my relatives, and all worldly things to learn yoga. I have made a firm resolve. Only when I become a yogi, will I return to my country. If not, I shall die in India."

I felt great love for Mr. Massac. At this time, I was no longer teaching any asana, pranayama, or meditation directly. My disciples were able to provide that instruction. Despite that, I taught him a little about postures and pranayama. After listening closely, Mr. Massac said to me, "I have heard that a true guru can give instruction through shaktipat (an energetic transmission), which quickly puts the disciple on the road to yoga. Guruji, please give this child shaktipat. It is not right for Indian gurus to give true yogic instruction only to other Indians. Please, do not scorn me as foreign and unholy."

I had known about shaktipat for many years. It was the yogic initiation given me by my guru. The yogic scriptures say that this initiation should only be given to a true and holy disciple of the highest caliber. A few months before, I had heard that several Indian gurus were publicly bestowing shaktipat and was greatly surprised by this. In this moment with Mr. Massac, I was faced with a dilemma. I had many loyal disciples but had not given shaktipat to any of them. While sincere, Mr. Massac had not proven himself a deserving candidate. Yet he was also correct that a student should not be denied simply because of being a foreigner. No matter what I might say, he would interpret my refusal this way.

In that moment, I felt this situation must be God's will. So I stopped thinking about it, and gave him the instructions preliminary to shaktipat. Afterward, I taught him a little about mudras (advanced energetic yoga practices) and a few other things. Finally, I told him to always chant the mantra Ram and showed him how to repeat it.

Being a foreigner, the Ram mantra was new to Mr. Massac. After hearing my instruction, his face turned serious and he asked, "Who is Ram? Why should I repeat his name? Being unfamiliar, I have no faith in chanting it." I made an effort to explain that Ram is a name of God, which one chants repeatedly to purify the mind. I *told him that this Ram mantra arises from the sound (nada) of the Infinite. Only when he hears this sound through the practice of yoga will he understand why I am instructing him to repeat it. Thereafter, I ended, "Whatever you like to chant, chant it."*

Within a few days, Mr. Massac returned having found a kootir (hut) in which to practice. I gave him the name of Shubhadarshan, initiated him in shaktipat, and he started his yoga sadhana as previously instructed. Some weeks later, Shubhadarshan came to pay his respects. He said, "Guruji, I ask forgiveness for the stupidity I showed in not wanting to repeat the Ram mantra. Truly, this Ram mantra has filled me with astonishment. Now I clearly understand why you say it arises from the Infinite. This deep, essential truth of yoga has not come through the strength of my study. It has been revealed to me by the strength of experience."

A year later he visited again. I motioned to him, "My son, Shubhadarshan, come sit. Tell me, are you still repeating the Ram mantra?" He laughed and replied in Hindi, "Gurudev, each cell and every hair of this body is full of the Ram mantra. I, on my own, from the moment of getting up, repeat Ram Ram Ram continuously. I hope you have no objections to my chanting of Ram, because it happens spontaneously."

Truly, this is an experience of yoga sadhana. An aspirant may be from any community, or belong to any religion, or come from anywhere the world over, but when their prana rises up these yogic mantras automatically spill out of their mouth.

The word shaktipat means "descent of the power." As a divine benediction, the experience appears to be quite similar to the way a Christian might report being touched by God or moved by the Holy Spirit. In yoga, the word shaktipat is also used to describe an energetic transmission from guru to disciple that is meant to jumpstart a disciple's yoga sadhana. At the time of the events narrated in this story, Dr. Massac was a single man in his early twenties. The sentiment he expresses to Swami Kripalu when describing his departure from his home country and resolve to "become a yogi" or "die in India" has strong renunciate overtones. SK responds by initiating him into a renunciate level practice of anahat nada.

Mystique surrounds the phenomenon of shaktipat. This story suggests there are two parts of the initiation as conveyed by SK. First, there is a body of practical instruction. It seems certain from my studies that Massac was instructed in the yogic technique of surrender, which enables a student to turn their mind-based will over to a higher power. If I am correct, this would be entirely consistent with the glossolalia research mentioned above, which characterizes those speaking in tongues as experiencing a subjective loss of self-control. Once Massac had secured a place to practice, the instruction was followed by an initiation ritual that gave him a new name and permission to commence practice. As warranted, his progress on the path of anahat nada is swift.

Lauture Massac, PhD is a clinical psychologist licensed and practicing in California. Yoga and meditation are integral elements in the professional approach he offers those wanting to experience holistic health and embark upon a journey of self-discovery. The events in this story occurred in 1970, which confirms that Dr. Massac was the first of SK's students to receive shaktipat initiation. This is a remarkable outcome for a western youth traveling to India to find a guru.

THE WOMEN AND THEIR DEAREST TREASURE

Swami Kripalu was born in the Indian state of Gujarat, which was home to a flourishing Hindu religious culture and Shaivite yoga lineage in the first ten centuries of the Common Era. The yoga lineage fell into decline with frequent raids by Muslim invaders, who killed its priests and plundered its network of shrines including the magnificent Somnath temple in 1026. It all but disappeared when Gujarat fell under the control of the Mughal Empire, which sanctioned an administrative policy of social and economic discrimination against anyone not subscribing to the state religion of Sunni Islam. Mughal rule would continue until 1756, when the colonizing British took control of the country. It is against this historical backdrop that SK tells this story.

> *Once in a small Indian city, fear was everywhere. The residents were Hindu, and the army of a powerful Muslim king surrounded the city. It seemed certain they would all be slaughtered. The army had appeared quickly with no warning. There was no time to get*

military help. As a result, the residents were totally at the mercy of the Muslim ruler.

Perhaps he would only demand their wealth and then leave. That was their hope. This thought was at least tolerable, as wealth can be replaced. But if the king turned his soldiers loose on the city with violence, rape, and a forced choice between religious conversion and death, everyone would suffer greatly.

The Muslim king knew the city had no army. It was defenseless and completely encircled. No one could escape without his approval. He considered allowing his soldiers to pillage the city, rewarding them with whatever they wanted. But he wasn't an uneducated brute. Born into a royal and religious family, he had been taught morality and fairness, not cruelty and fanaticism.

After the king had thought deeply about what to do, he announced his decision. He would permit his soldiers to rob the city of its wealth. But no women or children should be harmed. Moreover, to protect the women, he would let them leave the city before the army entered. In addition, each woman could carry one bundle on her head, so no mother or widow would find herself penniless. They could carry out anything they wanted—coins, costly jewelry, expensive clothes, family treasures, whatever they chose— but only one bundle.

The king sent his messengers into the city with the news. "Our army will enter the city tomorrow morning and take whatever we like. All the women can leave, but they must be gone by mid-morning. Every woman may carry one bundle on her head with anything she wants to save, but just one bundle. If the men choose to resist, we will fight with them."

At dawn, several thousand women were already lined up to leave the city carrying bundles on their heads. The king stayed true to his word. He unblocked the main road to allow the women to leave unmolested. Unbeknownst to anyone, the king himself was watching the procession. Very soon the king grew puzzled. All the women, even aged grandmothers, carried one huge bundle on their heads. The bundles weighed so much that their legs were buckling. The procession moved slowly because no one could walk far without resting.

The king thought to himself, "Not even gold and jewelry can weigh so much. What is it that all these women are carrying? Maybe it's a unique treasure found only in this area of the world. Perhaps I was mistaken in my decree? I better look into this."

The king made his appearance and commanded, "Everyone stop walking and put down your bundles." Up to now, the women's fear had greatly lessened. Terror again struck them as it seemed the king was taking back his promise and might order his army to harm them. But the women were helpless and had to follow his order.

"Untie each bundle," the king demanded in a loud voice. Everyone complied, and the king was astonished. There was no gold, no jewels, no money or pearls or expensive clothes in any of the bundles. All the women had willingly left these things back in their homes for the soldiers to take.

What then was in the bundles? There were children, helpless old men, ailing husbands, injured brothers, and sons old enough that they might be killed as men. The king asked the crowd, "How are these your most valuable items?" The women were fearful and remained silent. No one dared answer the king. Finally, a woman stepped forward to speak who was old enough to feel as if she had nothing to fear in losing her life.

"Oh great king," she said. "The dharma in which we were raised taught us how to love and serve our husbands, our children, our parents, and our grandparents. Yes, we regard them as priceless possessions. They are the all-in-all of our lives. They are our true wealth—not gold, silver, diamonds, or pearls. This is our religion, our sacred duty, our path to Almighty God, our pilgrimage to the Truth. We are simply practicing the holy dharma of our womanhood."

This answer plunged the king into deep thought. How could he plunder these people, when such love and service existed among them? He saluted the old woman for her forthright answer. With a single order, he turned his obedient army of soldiers away from the city's entrance, returning to his country without taking any act of aggression upon the helpless people.

This story affirms the value of familial love and suggests that a yogi should cherish the well-being of loved ones more than wealth. The story's positive outcome reinforces this message by showing how a person embodying the yogic practice of *love in the family* gains a nobility of character that will be recognized and bring unexpected good fortune. Another of those cultural values is religious tolerance. It is noteworthy that Swami Kripalu does not portray the Muslim king or his soldiers as unprincipled or bad people, but instead emphasizes their thoughtfulness and obedience.

THE MARRIAGE OF DIVARKA AND KALPALATA

Swami Kripalu taught that genuine love always expresses itself in service. When necessary, that includes a willingness to make personal sacrifices for the well-being of one's beloveds. These two themes of service and sacrifice appear often in this poignant story.

Once there was a young man named Divarka, whose parents had died when he was just a child. Shortly after his eighteenth birthday, his two uncles called him to their sides and said, "Divarka, it's time for you to get married. We've found a bride for you."

Divarka sat silently with downcast eyes. A minute passed before he spoke in a quiet but questioning voice. "I know you both only want what's best for me. You've raised me. You've educated me. Recently you've helped me obtain a job. But wouldn't it be best to wait until I'm older and more established before marrying?"

"We agree with you," his uncles said. "It would be better to wait, but we like this girl named Kalpalata very much. A few years from now, we may not be able to find someone with such good character." Divarka agreed and three days later he was married.

Divarka liked his new wife very much and was impressed by the good qualities evident in her thoughts, speech, and behavior. "Uncles," he said a short time later. "You made a wise choice for me. Kalpalata is a pearl of a woman. She has transformed my life." Divarka labored diligently in the shop of a successful food merchant. Kalpalata managed their home and household. Two years passed happily and they were joined by a son. Five years into their marriage, Divarka and Kalpalata had become one, their hearts resonating like two notes in perfect harmony. While their little family didn't live in luxury, they had what was needed and felt rich with the wealth of love.

Then tragedy struck. There was a fire in the shop and most of the inventory was lost. For two months, Divarka worked without pay as his employer struggled to reopen but the effort failed and the doors of the shop were closed. Divarka searched everywhere for work but no one was hiring. The family had no savings beyond a bag of rice. Kalpalata never complained. Instead, she worked secretly on the side. Doing laundry, she was able to earn a few rupees to keep their son from starving. For a time Divarka and Kalpalata had a little grain each day to eat, but they couldn't afford a vegetable to go with it.

Soon the bag of rice was empty, but Divarka's efforts to find another job remained fruitless. Weeks passed and one day Divarka asked his wife, "Tell me the truth. When was the last time you've eaten?" Kalpalata laughed and said "I've always wanted to do a long fast and there is no need to worry about me," but Divarka could tell it was a false laugh. Tears rolled down his face and Kalpalata wiped them away with her sari. "Don't lose heart," she said, "I am certain that you will not only obtain work but that we'll be better off because of this."

Divarka received consolation from Kalpalata's words, but she was not yet done speaking. "Do you believe me?" she asked. Divarka suffered a great loss in his childhood. As a result, he had never been a man of faith. When he didn't respond, Kalpalata pressed him for an answer, "Divarka, I want to know if you believe!" At that moment, a tiny spark of faith ignited in Divarka's heart. Looking his wife in the eyes he responded, "Yes, I believe." "Then listen to me," Kalpalata said. "My gold jewelry is worth 2000 rupees. Sell it and open a small shop."

Divarka was shocked. Kalpalata's jewelry was a family heirloom given by her deceased parents. If they ever had a daughter, it would be needed as her dowry. "How could I sell your jewelry? I'll think it over and tell you tomorrow." "No," Kalpalata said. "There is nothing to think about. Faith must be acted upon. The time to start a shop is now, while the needs of people are going unmet. For the sake of our family, sell the jewelry. After you become successful, you can replace it."

Divarka agreed. Within three months, his tiny rented shop was prospering. Soon he was able to buy the building, and before too long had to build two new rooms to handle his growing grocery business. Two years later, Kalpalata gave birth to a healthy daughter. Divarka approached the rich man who had purchased her jewelry and was able to buy back every piece. Divarka treated his customers well, and always helped those who had fallen upon hard times. Along with becoming a successful merchant, Divarka had become a man of faith.

Many happy years went by before tragedy struck again. Kalpalata's mind began to fail her. Her condition worsened until she didn't speak anymore. Sitting like a stone withdrawn into herself, she remained in a state that was neither conscious nor unconscious. Eventually she lost control of her bodily functions. Divarka passed on his business to his son, now married, so he could sit with Kalpalata every day. All his time was spent in keeping her fed and bathed. Each morning, he dressed her. Each evening, he put her to bed. Almighty God is love, and service his means to purify us all.

Divarka's friends were touched by his devotion to his wife but nonetheless gave him their unsolicited advice. "Divarka," they said. "Place Kalpalata in an asylum. She can live there peacefully under the supervision of doctors and you can have your life back. You will go mad yourself if you keep living like this." Divarka was a rich man now, and each of his friends had someone for him to marry, someone in their own family willing to share in his wealth. Finally, his closest friend approached him. "Divarka," he said. "Enough is enough. Your life has become miserable. Make arrangements for Kalpalata's care and remarry anyone you want."

"I can't do that," Divarka replied, speaking deeply from his heart. "Kalpalata is the reason I'm successful. She never abandoned me, even during my darkest moments. She's still the same Kalpalata to me, despite her illness. It would be despicable to abandon her now, when she needs me the most." His friend left, and saw to it that no one gave him this advice again.

When Kalpalata left her body, Divarka's concern for the world died with her. All of his attention had been focused on her care for so long that only an open space remained. Having lived a rich life as a man of faith, Divarka was ready to pursue the spiritual life with undivided focus.

Renunciate spiritual paths often characterize marriage as arising from the sexual instinct, fraught with gender differences and conflicts, and destined to turn into an unfulfilling power struggle. In this and other teaching stories, Swami Kripalu portrays marriage in a positive light as a natural expression and means for both partners to develop selfless and ennobling qualities. When Kalpalata dies, Divarka's future happiness is not dependent on obtaining the human companionship of a second wife. His fulfilling marriage with Kalpalata has prepared him to enter the final stage of a householder's life and seek the higher love of divine union.

THE NATURE OF A YOGI

The human tendency to look outside and engage in what Swami Kripalu called *fault finding* is deeply ingrained in most of us. To grow beyond it, a great effort must be made to replace our default pattern of criticizing others with the willingness and ability to see ourselves and our shortcomings clearly.

To reflect on the character of a true saint is a subtle form of meditation. Once a group of students went on a pilgrimage with their guru. After traveling several days on foot, they arrived at the holy site late in the evening, joining many other pilgrims who were likewise gathering. Night quickly fell, and since it was summer everyone simply laid down on the ground to rest.

It so happened the guru awoke at two o'clock. The full moon had risen in the sky, and he sat up to gaze at a pious and inspiring sight. The moonlight was illuminating the white clothing of thousands of pilgrims sleeping peacefully on the ground.

Hearing the faint noise of his guru rising, his foremost disciple also sat up. Looking about he whispered, "Guruji, look at all these people. Like us they have come for pilgrimage, but they have fallen asleep. Only you and I are awake to the solemn beauty of this moment." Hearing the pride reflected in this statement, the guru responded, *"My son, I've taught you that the nature of all great yogis is to want to remove the blemishes of their own character. But a yogi must also be quick to see the good in others. Right now, you are only seeing the shortcomings of your fellow pilgrims, which is blinding you to the fact that only a few minutes ago both you and I were sound asleep. This kind of arrogance will hinder your growth."*

The guru let a few moments pass so his teaching could be received. Then he ended their conversation, "But all of this is my fault for waking you up before you had sufficient sleep. Lie back down now and complete your rest. When you rise in the morning, be a true yogi who is quick to acknowledge his own faults and always affirms the highest in others."

Yogic aspirants who make the effort to progress along the path of character building will eventually confront an amplified version of the ordinary tendency to judge others. This is the well-known pitfall of spiritual pride. Exalting one's self and condemning others is never the way forward. In this story, that teaching is not just spoken by the guru. It is reflected in his saintly character, which SK urges us to meditate upon.

APPENDIX 3
INSTRUCTIONAL HANDOUTS

These are the instructional handouts included here.

- Becoming the Well-Wisher of All
- Breathe Your Way into Meditation
- Witness Meditation
- How to Do a Mantra Japa Retreat
- Mantra Meditation
- Inner Sound Meditation
- How to Chant Om
- Swami Kripalu on Karma Yoga

BECOMING THE WELL-WISHER OF ALL

Some forms of meditation are designed to open the heart and cultivate positive states like empathy, compassion, and forgiveness. The regular practice of these techniques is known to foster emotional healing and eventually lead to genuine feelings of happiness and joy. The best-known example of this type of meditation is the Buddhist practice of metta or lovingkindness. The below technique is a similar form of meditation that comes from the yoga tradition as referenced in chapter 12.

1. *Find Your Sweet Spot.* Close your eyes and take several relaxing breaths to center yourself in your body. Focus your awareness on your chest and see if you can locate your emotional sweet spot. This is your heart-center, a tender place beneath all your toughness and defensiveness. You may find your sweet spot tinged with sadness, or encounter uncomfortable feelings of vulnerability, anger, or grief. If possible, relax into these feelings and find your way to rest in the heart space.

2. *Start with Yourself.* Bring your attention to yourself. Then begin the process of wishing yourself well by inwardly and silently repeating the following prayer.

> May I be happy.
> May I be healthy.
> May I be safe from inner and outer harm.
> May I know the deep ease of wellbeing that is my true nature.
> May I be free of all suffering.

3. *A Loved One.* Bring your attention to someone close to you and wish them well by inwardly and silently repeating the following prayer.

> May you be happy.
> May you be healthy.
> May you be safe from inner and outer harm.
> May you know the deep ease of wellbeing that is your true nature.
> May you be free of all suffering.

4. *An Acquaintance.* Bring your attention to a neutral person and wish them well by inwardly and silently repeating the same prayer.

5. *A Person of Challenge.* Bring your attention to a person with whom you have some degree of difficulty and wish them well by inwardly and silently repeating the same prayer.

6. *Return to Yourself.* Bring your attention back to yourself. Take a moment to really notice how you are feeling. Close your practice by once again wishing yourself well by inwardly and silently repeating the prayer. Stretch in any way that feels good to establish yourself in your normal, embodied awareness before moving on to whatever is next for you.

Anyone can become a well-wisher—whether man or woman, young or old, rich or poor. If you aspire to tread the path of meditation, become the well-wisher of everyone. You will know you have truly progressed in your practice when there is no enmity in your heart for anyone.

BREATHE YOUR WAY INTO MEDITATION

Today's researchers are proving what yogis have known for millennia. Conscious breathing is the key to unlock your hidden potential to manage stress, regulate emotions, and access higher states of awareness. Here's a simple protocol based on what yoga calls ujjayi and dirgha pranayama that relaxes the body, soothes the nervous system, and quiets monkey-mind to ease your way into a meditative state. While learning it, you may want to dedicate ten minutes or more to practice. Once you've got the knack, just a few minutes of conscious breathing will be enough to internalize your focus and prepare you for postures or meditation, as referenced in chapter 13.

1. *Take Your Seat.* Adjust your sitting position to make the body comfortable. Press the sitting bones down, slightly tuck the chin, and lift through the crown of your head to elongate the spine. Close the eyes to facilitate inner focus.

2. *Find the Breath.* Tune into the breath and take a minute to simply notice how you are already breathing. Then locate the spot in the torso where you feel the flow of breath most acutely. As you watch the breath move in and out, invite this spot to gradually soften, facilitating an easy movement of the belly and diaphragm.

3. *Make the Breath Audible.* Slightly contract the back of the throat, allowing the friction of the breath against the glottis to make a sound like the rise and fall of waves against the beach. Making this sound (ujjayi pranayama) provides a way to closely monitor the quality of the breath. Allow the sound of your breath to be a soothing point of focus that anchors the mind in the sensation of breathing.

4. *Pendulum Breath.* As you sustain this sounding breath, a natural urge will arise to smooth the breath out. Let that happen by shifting between in-breaths and out-breaths as smoothly as possible. As the inhale completes, consciously relax the muscles of the chest. As the exhale completes, conscious relax the abdomen and belly. Surround the breath with a sense of ease and non-hurry. Instead of trying to breathe deeply, which tends to create tension, let the breath grow long and smooth, filling the lungs from bottom to top. You may find your breath flowing like a pendulum, with a relaxing pause as it changes direction. Sustain this breath for several minutes, drinking in its revitalizing power.

5. *Let Go into Belly Breathing.* As your next inhale completes, let go of any control of the breath. Watch as the breath rebalances, and you'll find your body naturally moving into belly breathing, where the movement of the diaphragm effortlessly brings air in and out. This is a body-based breath that does not require any mental monitoring. Once this new breath pattern establishes itself, you are ready to shift focus and practice yoga postures or engage any meditation technique.

> *In order to overcome distraction, the practice of yogic breathing is extremely useful. Its regular practice prior to meditation aids concentration and generates feelings of deep peace. Both of these greatly hasten one's progress. Whoever relies on the breath has obtained a key to yoga, as the seed of pranayama (yogic breathing) will invariably grow into the tree of self-realization.*

WITNESS MEDITATION

One of the primary benefits of meditation is gaining a greater understanding of how our minds work. Many mental patterns and much of our habitual self-talk perpetuate a state of anxiety and suffering, but it is not easy to see these patterns clearly, which is the first step in letting them go. This is a technique that increases self-awareness by teaching you how to objectively and non-reactively witness the activity of your own mind. It is one part of SK's approach to character building detailed in chapter 17.

1. *Take Your Seat.* Adjust your sitting position to make the body comfortable. Press the sitting bones down, slightly tuck the chin, and lift through the crown of your head to elongate the spine. Close the eyes to facilitate inner focus.

2. *Come into Belly Breathing.* See the prior handout for complete instructions.

3. *Follow the Breath.* Bring your attention to the highly-sensitive tip of the nostrils. Anchor your awareness there, simply watching and feeling the movement of air as it flows in and out of the nostrils. By sustaining this one-pointed focus, the mind will grow both relaxed and highly concentrated. For several minutes, simply follow the breath at the nostrils, allowing your attention to be singular and your awareness to grow laser-like.

4. *Become the Witness.* When concentration is established, gradually broaden out the scope of your awareness to include the full spectrum of sensations, feelings, and thoughts passing through you. Be intimate with the flow of your inner experience. See clearly, feel fully, resting in the state of non-judgmental observation that Kripalu Yoga calls Witness Consciousness.

5. *Investigate.* Whenever the mind drifts off into thought or story, come back to the breath and reestablish your focus. Notice whatever topic, stream of thought, or feelings pulled you out of witness consciousness. What does this have to teach you?

6. *Let Go of All Technique.* End your meditation by dropping any effort to focus the mind or understand your experience. Dropping all techniques, come into effortless being. Rest there until the end of session.

Unless a seeker studies the workings of his own mind, he will never find peace. Self-observation is the tool to mine the treasure of mind. One cannot obtain the capacity of self-observation all of a sudden. It must be learned gradually and there is a need for constant practice. But the effort will prove worthwhile, as self-observation is the source of all progress on the spiritual path.

HOW TO DO A MANTRA JAPA RETREAT

Here are Swami Kripalu's instructions on how to prepare for and successfully complete a self-guided mantra japa retreat as referenced in chapter 19.

Along with their regular worship (the daily practice of japa), a mantra yogi periodically retreats from their usual duties to renew their mantra anusthan (systematic and persistent practice). There are guidelines to follow when doing this.

Find a pious and private place to practice. This might be as simple as temporarily emptying a room in your house, but it is best if you have a secluded place completely free for your use. In India, it is not unusual to see this practice being performed outside under the canopy of a large tree.

Make practical arrangements that enable you to eat moderately. This is necessary for the body and mind to remain comfortable while doing a lot of japa. It is not advisable to fast as that is likely to lead you to recite the food mantra: "I haven't eaten, I haven't eaten, I haven't eaten." A moderate or scant diet is best.

Decide on the number of recitations that you will perform. Traditionally that means many thousands of times, but you can set any number.

For the duration of your mantra anusthan, live very simply. Protect your mental steadiness by remaining alone. Only engage in essential talking. Brothers do not need to shave. Sisters can forego their cosmetics. This is not a time for looking beautiful. That concern will take you in a different direction. In India, mantra anusthan is considered a time of upavasa, which means to sit close and expose yourself to God without artifice.

Each mantra belongs to a specific deity. Do some ceremony to invoke Its presence to begin the anusthan. Then each time you take your seat for japa, enter back into that presence, feeling as if the Lord in that form sits before you. It is useful to have an altar with a picture or statue of the deity to express that reality. However, one should not worry if such things are not available. Love does not need any external supports.

Just pronouncing the words of the mantra is not enough. You also have to absorb your mind by reciting the mantra with great feeling and love. Doing this will introvert the mind and all sorts of thoughts, feelings, and images will come up from the unconscious. Scenes from the past, imaginings of the future, many different things will come before you as you become inwardly quiet and intent upon your japa. If you have a statue or picture, you can open your eyes and gaze upon it to bring your attention back to the mantra and purpose of your practice. Use this image to remove any distracting images and renew your focus and inspiration.

Mantra recitation is not the worship of an image or idol. It is the worship of the hidden and unseen Spirit. Yet a person reciting mantra with great love and feeling may experience the deity coming alive. They may see the eyes and lips of the image on their altar moving, have heavenly inner visions, or find the Lord has come physically into their presence to bless or guide them. These are the private experiences of bhakti yoga – there is no place for logic in them. A practitioner should remain aware that all of this is happening in response to their strong mental focus and feelings of devotion. Consider them personal revelations. Don't make the mistake of seeing them as meant for others.

A second ceremony is performed to complete the anusthan. First the deity is thanked for its presence. In India, food is then offered to saints, swamis, or those in need in accordance with your financial capacity. In some way, offer back any benefits gained from the practice as a gift to others.

These are general guidelines. For mantra anusthan to be effective, japa has to be done in a quiet place. The mantra has to be recited with awareness and love. It has to be accompanied by moderation in diet. Beyond that, do your mantra anusthan wisely and tailor your practice in the specific ways most suitable to you.

MANTRA MEDITATION

The technique of quieting the mind by inwardly repeating a word or phrase appears in all the world's wisdom traditions. It is fully expressed in the eastern practice of mantra meditation and the Western practice of contemplative prayer. Both use a "sacred word" to center, calm, and eventually step beyond the limits of the mind. Along with a positive meaning, the chosen word should have a soothing sound, as both contribute to the power of this technique.

The instructions below use the word "peace" proven by Herbert Benson, MD, to elicit the relaxation response fundamental to stress management. While a mantra is commonly considered a word or phrase that gets repeated constantly to occupy the mind, that's a different practice called mantra japa or "recitation." This is a subtler technique that uses one thought—the only-when-necessary repetition of the word peace—to remove all other thoughts from the mind as explained in chapter 19. This brings you into moments of silence and stillness where it's possible to know the peace that passes all understanding.

1. *Take Your Seat.* Adjust your sitting position to make the body comfortable. Press the sitting bones down, slightly tuck the chin, and lift through the crown of your head to elongate the spine. Close the eyes to facilitate inner focus.

2. *Come into Belly Breathing.* See prior handout on page 316 for complete instructions.

3. *Breath Assisted Repetition.* As the breath flows naturally in and out, gently introduce the word "peace" into your awareness as a symbol of your intention to quiet the mind and experience inner peace. At first, you are likely to find yourself inwardly saying the word "peace" as the breath flows in, and saying the word "peace" again as the breath flows out. Let this link between the breath and the repetition of the word "peace" continue as the flow of thought through the mind gradually slows down.

4. *Repetition Without Support.* When the mind has noticeably slowed, let go of any link between the breath and the word. Allow your focus to shift from the individual thoughts passing through the foreground of the mind to the deep backdrop of awareness in which all sensations, feelings, images, memories, reflections, internal commentary and cognitions arise and pass away. As your awareness expands, the space between the thoughts grows apparent and the mind can open up.

5. *Return to The Word*. Whenever the thinking mind comes back in and you find distracted or lost in story, break the flow of thought by mentally saying the word "peace." Do this gently by simply re-introducing the word and notion of repeating it when needed. Re-center yourself, shift your attention from foreground to background, and allow your awareness to grow spacious. It is fine for periods of time to pass in which you entirely forget that you are repeating the word "peace." The objective is not to repeat the word but rather to learn to rest in moments of inner peace and spiritual receptivity. During these moments of stillness and transcendent awareness, trust that you are being informed by the cosmic mind and its profound creativity and ordering intelligence.

6. *Transition Gently*. At the end of your meditation period, sit quietly for a few minutes. This transition time is important, as it allows the psyche to return to its normal orientation. It also supports you in bringing the peace of your meditation back into your daily life. When you are ready to move on to the next thing, take a deep breath and open your eyes.

> *The Sanskrit word mantra in a derivative of the word manas which means "to think." Whatever we think in our mind is a mantra. When we think haphazard thoughts, we are repeating a very ordinary mantra. Done with great concentration of mind, a mantra has the power to transform every cell of your body and synapse of the mind.*

INNER SOUND MEDITATION

Many of the world's wisdom traditions include an approach to meditation based on inner listening. In the yoga tradition, this is an advanced technique done after a middle-tier technique like mantra meditation has rendered the mind still and quiet as explained in chapter 19. A practitioner who has found a way to enter the world of inner sound can do this technique on its own as instructed below.

1. *Take Your Seat.* Adjust your sitting position to make the body comfortable. Press the sitting bones down, slightly tuck the chin, and lift through the crown of your head to elongate the spine. Close the eyes to facilitate inner focus.

2. *Come into Belly Breathing.* See prior handout on page 316 for complete instructions.

3. *Listen to Outer Sounds.* With the eyes closed, begin your meditation by taking a few minutes to simply listen. As you become acquainted with the soundscape surrounding you, note any sounds that are particularly loud or distant. Attend to these sounds first by listening to them closely. Then one-by-one attend to softer and closer sounds. Do not hurry this process, giving yourself time to acknowledge the full spectrum of sounds in your outer environment, which is likely to include distant sounds like highway noise or wind in the trees, and close sounds like the hum of household appliances and the movement of your breath.

4. *Smoothly Shift to Inner Sounds.* Inner sound meditation is meant to shift awareness from the external world of gross sense-perception to an internal world in which hearing turns inward and begin to notice subtle sounds that are easily overlooked and ignored. Learning how to activate your hearing faculties by progressively attending to loud, then soft, then subtle outer sounds is one of the secrets of this technique. Once acknowledged and thereby normalized, these sounds lose much of their power to command and distract attention. Only then can effective inner listening begin.

5. *Listen to Inner Sounds.* Listening inward, you are likely to hear the sounds of the physical body engaged in its work. First, you may hear the breath moving in and out of the lungs. Then you may hear your heartbeat and sounds associated with blood moving through the circulatory system. Listening intently, you may discover a layer of higher-pitched sounds arising from the activity of the nervous system. At this point, you are poised to enter a range of meditative states that can reveal the presence of a deeper and unsuspected soundscape.

6. *Deepen Your Listening.* Those new to this technique may find it helpful to temporarily press the ear flaps closed with the thumbs to eliminate all but the loudest of outer noises. Closing the ears in this way also heightens the psychological sense of internalizing the awareness and attuning the auditory faculties to an inner world. Ear plugs may be used, but they are less effective. Remember, not everyone hears these inner sounds, especially at first. But those who feel called to stick with the practice may discover a layer of sounds beneath or behind those arising from the body and nervous system. Don't try to make anything happen. Simply be present to whatever you naturally experience.

7. *Attune to Inner Sounding.* Examine any inner sounds you encounter, noticing any changes or modulations. Listen closely to see if you can hear another even subtler sound behind it. Participate in the process, but don't try to control it. Instead, let your awareness follow the sounds as they shift and change. Notice if this results in you being drawn deeper and deeper into meditation.

8. *The Om Sound and Inner Light.* As your meditation time draws to a close, notice if you can hear any sound that seems steady or constant. It may start out as a high-pitched tone or ringing that is barely audible. If so, bring all of your awareness to bear upon that sound. Do not be afraid if it responds by growing louder, even to the point of roaring. At this point in the technique, whether you have heard any steady sound or not, you may begin to sense the presence of an inner light or see colors or geometric patterns. Or you may feel into the spiritual heart and encounter an abiding depth of love. If this occurs, let any of these attract your attention. Yoga teaches that inner sound (nada), inner light (jyoti), and spiritual love (prem) are closely related. Basking in love or light may enable you to more easily hear the Om vibration. If and when you hear the Om vibration, the yogic instruction is to allow your small sense of self to dissolve into the cosmic sound.

9. *Transition Gently.* End your meditation by dropping any effort to focus inward or understand your experience. Just sit quietly for a few minutes. This transition time is important, as it allows the psyche and senses to return to their normal orientation. When you are ready to end your meditation, take a deep breath and open your eyes. Stretch in any way that feels good, and consciously move on to the next thing.

In the early stages of yoga, the mind is multi-pointed and restless, running continuously after one object and then another. In the late stages of yoga, the mind is one-pointed and ready for absorption. Inner sound meditation is a method of attaining absorption by attuning to the audible expressions of the subtle sound current (nada). That is why the Hatha Yoga Pradipika instructs us to perform this meditation only after steadying the mind through other yoga techniques. While not for everyone, an accomplished yogi can come to know the essence of all existence through this method, which is beyond any particular form. This is why inner sound meditation will always remain a chief yogic technique.

HOW TO CHANT OM

This is an advanced mantra yoga technique given by Swami Kripalu for seasoned students wanting to experience depth meditation or move into the practice of anahat nada as explained in chapter 19.

The pranav mantra (Om) is reverenced by all yogic paths. On the householder path, the seed of Om is placed within a larger mantra. This is evident in Om Namah Shivaya, Om Namo Narayan, and Om Namo Bhagavata Vasudevaya. To chant just the seed mantra Om is very potent and considered too strong for householders. It is for this very reason that householders are given a longer mantra.

I will now give you a proven technique for practicing Pranav Japa. Sit in any comfortable position. Keep the body straight without straining. Stop the mind from wandering by becoming introspective and paying no heed to the external environment. The eyes may be closed or allowed to remain open. If kept open, the gaze should be steady. This technique is traditionally done with a harmonium but any musical instrument can be used.

Play middle C, listening attentively to pick up the pitch. Take a deep breath and chant a long Om, letting your mind become absorbed in the sound waves emanating all around you. Afterward, sit again silently.

Go up a fifth to G. Once again, listen to the pitch. Chant Om for as long as your breath lasts, concentrating on the sound waves and again become silent.

Go up to C one octave above the starting note and repeat.

Descend to G and repeat.

Return the middle C, where you begin, and repeat. You will have chanted Om a total of five times.

The mantra Ram can be chanted this way but there is a difference. The Om mantra is pronounced a single time in each breath. When chanting Ram, the mantra can be repeated rapidly as many times as possible: Ram, Ram, Ram. Other than this, the technique for both is the same.

If this practice is done daily, with a steady and attentive mind, for at least one repetition, every cell of your body and brain will be filled with peace and joy. If practice is gradually extended to a limit of one hour, you will be carried into divine experience.

SWAMI KRIPALU ON KARMA YOGA

The following excerpt does more than summarize the content of chapter 20. It provides detailed instruction on how to progress through the stages of karma yoga.

The Indian scriptures have been widely distributed in the West and everywhere the Bhagavad Gita's praises are sung. Yet its manner of expression is unusual and its message often not understood, even by those inclined to the spiritual life.

Upon close observation, we will see that no one can remain alive for a moment without action. Even if we sit perfectly still, our senses continue to operate. The eyes see outer or inner images. The ears register sounds. Inside the body the breath moves and we feel the many functions of life being carried on. All this activity agitates the mind and binds us to suffering. But inactivity is not an alternative available to us, as only a dead person can be considered truly inactive. This is why the Gita says that in order to master any type of yoga a student must begin by learning the lessons of karma yoga – the yoga of action.

Karma Yoga defines yoga as skillfulness in action. But before we can start acting skillfully, we must gain some action know-how. Doing good deeds that result in merit and avoiding bad deeds that result in downfall is a common religious idea. Karma Yoga is meant to take us beyond this ordinary religion by teaching us how to give up any sense of attachment to the results of our actions. This can only be done by adopting a certain mindset. A faith-oriented person dedicates his actions to the Lord. A reason-oriented person dedicates his actions to the welfare of others. Both walk a path of sacrificial action, purifying their motivation by offering their actions to the highest and abandoning attachment to its fruits.

While at first this may be difficult, it becomes simple with practice. We continue to discharge our duties, which are good actions worth taking. We refrain from evil actions, which are best avoided. Practically speaking the body needs food, so we act to obtain it. The mind needs security, so we act to remove insecurities. The inner being needs to evolve, so we act in ways that increase our energy and insight. Yet we perform all these actions with non-attachment and an attitude of pleasing the Lord or serving others. After taking action, we accept whatever the outcome may be. As we become steady in this discipline of karma yoga, we learn how to act without becoming excited by the prospect of success or fearful over the possibility of failure. Yogis who can maintain this quality of equanimity in their interactions develop skillfulness, often meet with success, and are quick to demonstrate mastery in life.

But even these non-attached and virtuous actions arise from the mind, which is conditioned by all our past experiences. This is why the path of karma yoga has another step. As long as there is an ego directing the actions, the sense of being the doer remains and binds us to suffering. Where dedicated action purifies the mind of self-centeredness, the next step aims to remove this sense of doership. A faith-oriented yogi ceases to consider himself the doer by affirming: "I do not perform voluntary actions. I perform only those actions the Lord does through me. I am not the actor. I am an instrument of the supreme spirit." Likewise, the reason-oriented yogi affirms: "I am the pure soul (atman) and unmoving witness. Nature is the active agent. I perform no actions on my own. While the body I live in may act, it is nature alone doing this work." Both relinquish the ego identification that makes them feel like the doer of the actions. They do not apply their will to force anything to happen, nor do they resist anything that wants to happen.

When there is no actor or ego, it can seem like nothing is left to instigate actions. Yet something is left that can only be found in practice. What remains is the natural action (sahaja karma) that springs directly from the spiritual source. To an outside observer these natural actions appear like any other actions, but they are totally unlike ordinary actions because they are not motivated by the mind's fears and desires. It is to differentiate the two that these natural actions are called by technical names including akarma karma (inaction in action), nishkam karma (action without desire), yajna karma (sacrificial action), and sharanagati karma (surrendered actions). These are all different labels for actions divorced from the will to act and thereby free of all the mind's polarities. A yogi who knows this true form of action experiences no disturbance or suffering despite all the actions taking place within his body and mind. Where mind-based actions bind us to suffering, these natural actions liberate a yogi from bondage.

These principles of karma yoga are useful in the meditation room as well as your daily life. Along with bringing mental steadiness, they will rouse the sleeping energy necessary to successfully conclude your spiritual or worldly work. I believe this is sufficient guidance for your contemplation of verse 2-48 of the Bhagavad Gita, which states: "Standing firm in yoga, do thy work, Oh Winner of Wealth (Arjuna), abandoning attachment to success or failure, for this evenness of mind is called yoga."

YOU MAY ALSO BE INTERESTED IN

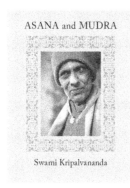

ASANA AND MUDRA SWAMI KRIPALVANANDA

"Swami Kripalu was a lightning bolt wrapped in an orange robe." —Richard Faulds

This book is addressed to practitioners of both the surrendered and willful paths of yoga. It describes the asanas that occurred to Kripalu spontaneously and gives detailed instructions on how to practice them. It also includes chapters on mudra, pranayama, and all the other components of yoga practice, as well as chapters on anatomy and physiology, psychology, and ayurvedic prescriptions for the healing of thirty diseases. It is truly an encyclopedia of yoga.

824 pages illustrated with 227 b/w photos. Considered by many to be Swami Kripalu's masterwork.

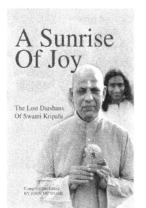

A SUNRISE OF JOY: THE LOST DARSHANS OF SWAMI KRIPALU COMPILED AND EDITED BY JOHN MUNDAHL

The life and impact of the greatest yogacharya of the 20th century

On May 20, 1977, Pan American flight 695 touched down at Kennedy Airport in New York City carrying a great treasure, not in gold or silver, but in the spiritual realm. A saint, revered by hundreds of thousands of people in India, had agreed to visit the US. This book tells the remarkable story of Swami Kripalu's life and his extraordinary stay in the US from 1977-81, when he broke his silence of many years and delivered more than 100 talks on a vast array of spiritual topics, most of which were published for the first time in this book.

FROM THE HEART OF THE LOTUS: THE TEACHING STORIES OF SWAMI KRIPALU COMPILED AND EDITED BY JOHN MUNDAHL

The teaching stories of Swami Kripalu—down-to-earth and transcendent

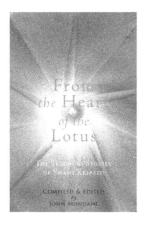

The Swami was fond of telling stories as a way of making his often subtle and surprising points. For example, in a parable about mind control, "The Demanding Daughter," we learn of a young spoiled woman who will only marry on the condition that she can find a husband who will allow her to strike him on the head seven times a day with her shoe.

Each story is set off by a particular yoga principle that the Swami illustrates through the story. Edited by John Mundahl who was a resident at the original Kripalu Yoga Ashram from 1977-81.

AVAILABLE FROM BOOKSELLERS EVERYWHERE
MONKFISH BOOK PUBLISHING • RHINEBECK, NEW YORK • MONKFISHPUBLISHING.COM

www.ingramcontent.com/pod-product-compliance
Lightning Source LLC
Jackson TN
JSHW082333240225
78877JS00002B/2